IRON FOOTPRINT FITNESS

Motivation Through Achievement

ANNE LARSON Ed.D

Iron Footprint Fitness is published to provide information relevant to physical activity participation with the understanding that it is not rendering legal, medical, or other professional services. Please consult with a physician or other expert before beginning any physical activity program. The expressed ideas are the opinion of Iron Footprint Fitness and results may vary.

Library of Congress Cataloging-in-Publication Data
Iron footprint fitness

ISBN: 0615720447

ISBN 13:   9780615720449

Library of Congress Control Number: 2012952455
Iron Footprint Fitness, Marina Del Rey, CA

To the best family a gal could wish for:
Thanks for endless backyard ball

To O-Man, Finnigan, Jakers, Lily-Hoo, and Lucky-Boy:
May you be blessed with health and a passion for play

To those of you wanting to start (or restart) an activity program,
or those of you wanting to get faster, stronger,
jump higher, throw farther...:
I hope this approach helps. I know you can do it!

CONTENTS

FOREWORD

Welcome!

Physical activity is my vocation, but mostly it's my love and me at my best. Yet like many, I get that motivation to engage can fluctuate and I've experienced the highs and lows of participation. I've hit game winners and made errors that caused a loss, I've won running road races and thrown up after finishing dead last in others, I've held powerlifting records but I've done panic dieting to lose weight for special events and for the record I miserably failed the gym class rope climb...

Through my teens I was a competitive swimmer. Good—not great. Never close to hitting elite times, but I sure loved the process how it fed my sense of accomplishment. At the suggestion of a coach, I kept a notebook of each day's workout. What a kick—indelible accomplishment. One notebook turned into two, turned into several, also turned into separate ones for my other sports, and yet another for my 'best-ofs.' At first I used my 'best-ofs' to track my fastest times for events or game statistics but then it became fun to make up 'events' to track like fastest time around the block and most combination sit ups – push ups in one minute. Admittedly, I haven't attempted that one in...decades!

Though with less detail, I continue to keep an eye on my 'performance,' and through the years amid moving across the country and back with stops in-between my notebooks are among the few keepsakes that have avoided the trash. Considering their meaning, I can't see parting with them, for especially during phases where my motivation ebbed due to hitting a performance plateau or batting slump, etc., capturing *something* about the process – *it wasn't fast but I did swim a total of 8000 yards at practice* - meant I could still enjoy a sense of accomplishment. The disappointment of lousy times or fielding errors aside, the process of notching was a rock to my motivation. At the least it was a distraction to poor performance in my 'formal' events–*I can't seem to go faster in the 100 freestyle but I improved my combination sit-ups – push-ups by 12*–that gave me hope all was not lost.

My nephew and niece have followed in the swimming footsteps of their parents (and their proud aunt) and I passed along the suggestion of keeping a notebook, which prompted me to dig my swimming ones out of the closet. As if each entry had just occurred, instantly my senses filled with the sights and sounds of being back at the pool. And, I admit, my pride boosted from reliving challenging practices and remembering races won.

Which made me wonder.

Sometimes it's harder to get motivated to be active than the activity/ workout itself because we get discouraged thinking we are not making gains, or have such a narrow view of what activity achievement is we hardly give ourselves a chance to realize success, or get dulled by a monotonous routine that has become 'too routine.' Maybe others would benefit as I have by tracking their activity and being able to 'see' all their success? Further, maybe this is how we ought to approach physical activity? Think about **all** the ways we can achieve, organize our engagement accordingly, then capture and showcase our achievement, both to snapshot our physical activity portfolio and have to sustain motivation.

Which reminded me that many of you have been so poorly served in activity it's no surprise your motivation suffers.

I don't take it for granted that I have been lucky along the way with opportunity, support and encouragement because it's been the polar opposite for so many of you. Not to presume, but none of us is motivated to do that in which we have realized limited success or feel incompetent. It's no surprise that so many have a pattern of re-starting activity programs more so than sustaining one.

Which inspired the idea of Iron Footprint Fitness.

Iron Footprint Fitness is an innovative approach to physical activity that introduces the multi-dimensional enterprise of engagement and offers a platform to foster resilient motivation by showcasing achievement within the enterprise's (strange sounding) categories of FitBASE, FitBUBBLES, and FitBESTS.

Iron Footprint Fitness transforms the dangerously narrow measure that typically gauges activity success by identifying engagement's generous potential for achievement, and describing how to capture it for display. The approach is universally adaptable to anyone regardless of previous experience in physical activity or level of proficiency, and free-of cost to adopt, but it isn't a gimmick or miracle. It won't take exertion's burn away, but it can ease the effort required to get to the gym or go for a run or play basketball at the park, then do the same the next day.

For those of you who struggle to stick to a physical activity routine or have felt only limited success, I hope you can use the approach to realize all that you DO achieve and grow your physical activity portfolio. For those of you who have experienced success, I hope it will inspire even greater achievement. Mostly I'm hoping Iron Footprint Fitness will foster your resilient motivation to sustain regular engagement. Your well-being matters! Notch on ...

IRON
FOOTPRINT
FITNESS

Motivation Through Achievement

PROLOGUE - GROUND RULES - WARM-UP

The nasty push/pull of physical activity.

At times we love it.

Can't wait to get outside—beautiful day. My Ipod is loaded and juiced, my legs feel great. I'm going 5 miles, not 4. Ahh, exhilarating, satisfying, calming, empowering.

But at other times we hate it, and the gremlins sing loud and strong.

Dread, petulance. But I know I need to do it, and I want arms that look like [insert celebrity name here]. It's soooooooooooooo good for us [said sarcastically], so good that I resent it. So good? I'll show you so good [we mutter to ourselves]. Why don't my arms look like [insert celebrity name here] yet?

So we negotiate our commitment.

I'm going easy today, but I swear I'm going to go hard tomorrow. I'm here, isn't that enough? I'm just doing arms today; I'll do legs tomorrow, along with back. I'm having dessert tonight. If the lot is full, I'm going home.

Then more petulance as we change clothes.

Kicking and screaming, pouting and scowling. Nothing feels right. I hate these shorts. It's so crowded in here. Who is that strange person? Why is it so cold? I hate the music! Who put the TV on that station? This bike never works!

Until we do it, and it's ...

> *Exhilarating,*
> *Satisfying,*
> *Calming,*
> *Empowering.*

Ahh, so it is. Serenely, we exhale. Take delight in our accomplishment of follow-through. Shoulders back, head up. Take pride in a good hurt. Notice the warm breeze on our face. Savor feeling refreshed and invigorated. Light on our feet. Traffic? What traffic? Wow! This is great. Can't wait to get back tomorrow.

Until tomorrow.

When the storm before the calm rages again. When the gremlins do their cruel best to invade our psyche like weeds in a garden and sap our intent. When exercise fatigue renders us comatose...

• • •

Nothing else impacts quality of life like physical activity. It has the unique power to foster vitality and vigor today and across the lifespan. Yet we sure can treat it like dirt.

For something so simple, uncomplicated, non-judgmental, reliable, and accessible ...

We vilify and taunt it.

For something that works whether we are short, tall, wide, narrow, knock-kneed, pigeon-toed, righthanded or lefthanded, skilled, clumsy, fast, experienced or novice ...

We disparage its generosity.

For something so valuable, so powerful, and so critical to our very well-being ...

We do our darndest to sabotage and undermine our regard and approach.

Well, that's not very nice. After all, it only wants to help. And anyway, we get it. We know it is good for us. We know we need to get activity every day. But we wish it were that simple. Some days we can't wait to get started, but other days, getting to the start is a battle, much less putting effort into the activity. The gremlins start singing and *they* creep in. The 'I'm too tired,' 'I bet the parking lot is full,' 'I don't have any clean gym clothes,' 'I forgot my lock.' The excuses, mind tricks played to talk ourselves out of going, and reasons conjured for why we shouldn't go.

And, boy, it sure becomes pretty easy to stay at home.

But then I feel guilty because I didn't go! Because I know I need to go and I do always feel great when I finish!

Ugh!

We hate to hate it and want to love it. So, how can we stop the gremlins, push back against the push/pull, quell the storm before the calm, reduce the stifling weight of exercise fatigue? How can we make it easier to simply, dare I say, just do it?

Resilient motivation.

Motivation that guards against the 'justs,' the negotiations that result in less than stellar gym efforts. Motivation that repels negative self-talk.

Motivation that fends off influences suggesting not to work out today.

Motivation that resists the temptation to stay on the couch in the warm/cool indoors.

Motivation that withstands long days at work, short nights of sleep, snarled traffic, and crowded gyms.

Motivation that pushes harder than the push/pull.

Motivation that doesn't feel the weight of exercise fatigue.

Motivation that is sag-resistant.

And, motivation that sustains a regular physical activity habit.

Okay, so how?

At its simplified essence, resiliency is part hope and part autonomy. So, to strengthen the resiliency of our physical activity motivation, we need to foster hope and autonomy specific to our physical activity engagement. Hope is about optimism, having a positive outlook, looking forward to something, and anticipating the best. Autonomy is about independence, self-sufficiency, and sovereignty.

So what can drive the development of these attributes specific to physical activity engagement?

Success!

As in realizing achievement. As in recognizing and acknowledging the gains we make and the results we obtain. For within achievement lies the realization that we *have* achieved and the anticipation that we *will continue* to achieve. Achievement also provides evidence of physical activity autonomy: we are strong, powerful, skilled.

And so it follows that our motivation to continue to engage stands strong and powerful. After all, success begets success begets success.

Which is why so many of us struggle to sustain a regular physical activity habit, and why it is so easy for the gremlins to commandeer our physical activity psyche.

We fail to recognize our successes because we fall prey to seeking narrowly framed, unrealistic goals.

We miss the gains we make while looking for the gains we are not going to find.

Whoa!

These two wrongs will never make a right, but more importantly, they set off a downward-spiraling chain reaction that can be difficult to stem. Frustration and discouragement follow over not realizing results that were unrealistic to begin with, with each landing sticky blows to our motivation to continue to engage. This opens the door to the nasty gremlins, and the chime of the push/pull becomes louder than our ability to talk over it. We stop going to the gym, we stop jogging, we stop taking the stairs. We stop our own push/pull because we can't overcome *the push/pull*, and we stop doing what uniquely can positively impact our well-being.

But the good news is that there is good news.

What follows is the launch of a concept about how to foster gremlin-resistant, resilient physical activity motivation through *accessing your multi-dimensional physical activity-related achievement by stamping your physical activity footprint, your **IRON FOOTPRINT.***

First, physical activity is an *enterprise* whose engagement ought to be considered accordingly. The complexity of engagement far surpasses the simple checkmark of 'Yes, I went to the gym today' or 'No, I didn't go to the gym today.' That doesn't provide a very compelling reason to go in the first place, as it doesn't provide purpose that we can dig into. It also doesn't nearly capture all the good the experience can yield. Nor is it visceral enough to increase the hope or autonomy that is essential to resilient physical activity motivation.

Related, the 'My legs are still fat' or 'My arms are still flabby' or 'I still don't have a six-pack' assessments that we typically use to gauge results wholly fail to allow us to acknowledge any gains we *have* made toward reducing body fat, or increasing muscle mass, or otherwise enhancing aspects of our physical self. For example, during a physical activity session we may bench press more weight than ever or run our fastest mile ever. Or we may have finally gotten up the nerve to take a new group fitness class. Or the session itself may have been a personal best for consecutive days of activity engagement.

Each of these is an achievement that ought to be identified, captured, and acknowledged!

See how this makes the 'Yes, I went to the gym today' or 'No, I didn't go to the gym today' or 'My legs are still fat' checkmarks and gauges of success we typically apply to engagement so thin and hollow, vacuous, and sorely inadequate?

And see how the typical engagement checkmarks and gauges of success serve to feed the gremlins?

The primary gist of **Iron Footprint Fitness** is to identify, acknowledge and showcase *any* physical activity achievement that is made (talk about growing hope and autonomy!) and to consider the achievement that can be identified from a broad perspective.

This requires that a platform be in place to accommodate, record, and capture the achievement.

And that platform is an icon that captures the whole of your physical activity footprint, your **Iron Footprint**: a graphic depiction of your physical activity achievement portfolio according to the dimensions that comprise the enterprise of physical activity engagement.

Barring complication, while some physical activity engagement is good, more is better. And given its unprecedented ability to positively impact our very well-being, we ought to strive to engage as much as possible. Our Iron Footprint ought to be as big, bad, loud, deep, steep, fat, thick, heavy, and wide as possible. For we build resilient motivation by watching our Iron Footprint grow, and grow our Iron Footprint as we build resilient motivation. Hope springs eternal as we relish the achievements we stamp, and stamp, and stamp. Autonomy is evidenced by improved indices of physical attributes: strength, endurance, skill execution, and group fitness class competence.

And, not to forget the gremlins, the blankety-blank-blank gremlins. Finally, their collective annoying voice is silenced. Their bottom-feeding antics have no nourishment. They shrivel into dust, for hope and autonomy trump their sorry !@#$%.

Important to note is that while you *don't* have to buy new workout clothes or sneakers, or a piece of exercise equipment, or an instructional DVD, this is not a gimmick that promises *fast, easy* results. Not nearly. You need to *commit* to engaging in activity *regularly* and with sufficient *intensity* to induce results. This means cardio exercise that gets your heart-rate into its training zone, weight training with weights heavy enough to actually build mass or endurance, AND motor skill practice to improve your proficiencies. More on this herein...

The devil is in the details, and what follows is the rest of the story, the filled-in blanks, the dotted i's and the crossed t's. The book is divided into five parts with each part performing a specific function to deliver concept to application and express the unique and distinguishing features of the approach. Part I introduces the dilemma of inconsistent engagement motivation and the Iron Footprint Fitness solution to the predicament. Part II follows by first, presenting the 'what's' of the concept and the 'why's' of how it has the ability to be a solution, then bridging application by describing the achievement contours of each engagement dimension along with activity suggestions and guidelines for how to create your achievement icon. Part III describes why approaching physical activity as Iron Footprint can be beneficial in greater depth, especially how creating and maintaining your achievement icon can foster motivation. Part IV offers a compilation of special-topic essays that guide your adoption of the approach and highlight its unique and distinguishing features. Part V explains the book's connection to the Iron Footprint Fitness website (ironfootprintfitness.com), which you gain access to as an added value to your purchase of this book. Included is an overview of the features of the website and instructions for how to gain membership. Last, three appendices offer additional aids to becoming familiar with and using the approach: Frequently Asked Questions and Definitions provide quick reference, templates provide formats to use to plan activity and create your Iron Footprint achievement icon, and a description of the approach's benefit to a wide-range of industry professionals explains its comprehensive potential.

You might notice that the key concepts of the approach are mentioned frequently throughout the book but from different perspectives. This is intentional 'spiraling,' or the revisiting of a previously discussed concept after additional information is 'scaffolded' (added to the mix). Admittedly, spiraling is a more appealing word to use than 'repeating' but the gist also differs. The point isn't to be rote or repetitious (or annoying) but to increase understanding by presenting key concepts amidst different scenery, unlike a 'one-and-done' approach. This way if we don't catch you from one angle hopefully we will from another.

For now, sit back, enjoy, and see you at the end.

PART I

THE DILEMMA AND A SOLUTION

Considering your relationship to physical activity:

Do you know you need to do it but struggle to do it?

Does your commitment to daily physical activity fluctuate?

Do you wish your motivation were more predictably consistent?

Have you purchased gym memberships or personal training time, only to not use either?

Do you feel guilty about your level of activity?

Do you feel that your physical activity self is underdeveloped (e.g., motor skills, strength, flexibility)?

Is formal exercise your sole form of physical activity?

Do you avoid certain physical activities because you lack confidence in your ability?

Are the types of physical activities you do limited for the same reason?

Do you consider yourself clumsy and uncoordinated?

Do you ever wonder how other people can have fun doing physical activity?

Have you had poor physical activity experiences as a child? Adolescent? Adult?

Considering your exercise routine:
> *Does your routine seem stale, uninteresting, or 'too routine'?*
> *If you go to a gym, do you only use a small percentage of the equipment available?*
> *Do you wish you knew more about fitness?*
> *Do you ever wonder what gains you are making?*
> *Do you get discouraged because you don't see results?*
> *Have you set resolutions to exercise more, only to fail to comply?*
> *Have you purchased exercise equipment, used it for a few days, then put it in storage or thrown it away?*
> *Do you find yourself approaching your workout from a 'just' perspective, as in 'Today I'm just going to do a little cardio' or 'Today I'm just going to do a few weights'?*

Any yeses?

Alienation from your physical self, lack of confidence in your physical activity ability, uncertainty about how to modify your routine, under-developed motor skills, physical activity participation that is limited to formal exercise, poor physical activity experiences growing up ...

If this characterizes your relationship to physical activity or your exercise routine, it's no wonder you struggle to sustain regular participation. Experiencing any one factor can significantly erode motivation, much less any combination of two or more.

You are not alone! Many of us have a relationship with physical activity that ebbs and flows, often ebbing more than flowing. As a fix, pocketbooks take the brunt of the push/pull. Gym memberships, time with personal trainers, home equipment, workout routine DVDs, and new workout clothes are purchased.

Short-term, the 'new' can provide a lift, and invigorate. But long-term, the 'new' isn't sustainable because it doesn't solve the root issue.

'Not having time' is a primary reason for inconsistent participation in physical activity, especially formal exercise, the most common form of physical activity engagement. No doubt we are busy, and among family, work, and other commitments, it's a challenge to squeeze physical activity into already jam-packed days.

But might there be an underlying issue for which 'busy' becomes the convenient reaction?

Disappointment caused by *not realizing success* is the culprit—especially the quick body transformation we are led to believe we should expect, but *don't* see.

Yet we keep trying to try.

For many, participation in physical activity is approached and assessed from a grossly narrow, one-dimensional perspective—solely considered for its formal exercise utility and as the gateway to the body we want. But we are also mindful of its goodness ("You need to exercise because it's good for you"), so inherently conflicted about both our motives and our goals, we attempt to dutifully (and perhaps resentfully) trek to the gym to get in our requisite cardio exercise or weight training. And while outwardly extolling the face value of its goodness, we think, "So what, if I still can't get into a pair of size 4 jeans or have abs that look like those on the *Men's Fitness* cover!"

And so we pursue the body transformation we are led to believe is easy and quick while resenting being told what to do ("You need to exercise!"), which—for even the most mature among us—can trigger exercise fatigue from the weight of the obligation we feel or adolescent-like rebellion. It is haphazard or effort-lite, with one foot figuratively in and one foot out, as we walk on the treadmill for the requisite time and complete a few sets of strength training. But when the promised, easy, immediate, radical transformation doesn't happen, motivation evaporates—toward which no amount of money thrown to the 'new' can remedy. As a self-preserving response to our perceived failure, we become 'busy,' but 'busy' is a disguise. What we are really avoiding is facing continued disappointment.

And so we stop trying to try.

But what if it were different? Wouldn't it be:

- *Relieving* to consistently look forward to your daily workout?
- *Fulfilling* to develop your physical activity profile as broadly as possible?
- *Gratifying* to actually 'see' the outcomes you derive from your physical activity participation?
  and
- *Fun* to have fun while doing physical activities?

Physical activity engagement brings with it the benefits of *Every Time* as well as the benefits of *Over Time*. Each time we engage in a physical activity we can reap a sense of satisfaction, stress reduction, and cognitive clarity, to name a few. Over time, if engagement is according to the protocol required to yield health protection, we can realize markers of well-being that preserve vitality and quality of life—healthy blood pressure, cholesterol level, body weight, and body composition. But these results take time, and because they are not immediately recognizable, we often don't realize the improvements we are making, and become discouraged because we think we are not making progress. (Although some body transformation can occur with due diligence [e.g., weight loss, muscle gain], it's not fast, nor without effort, nor instantly radical. Over time, yes; overnight, no. And change is felt before it is seen—we feel stronger before we see muscle definition. (More on the 'change process' is available for download at www.ironfootprintfitness.com).

This is not your fault! Because we don't know differently, because much about how we feel toward physical activity stems from deepseated roots, and because much of what we come to learn about physical activity is merely urban-legend myth, this is how we come to regard our approach to engagement and how to consider achievement.

But what if there were a different way? What if we could transform our approach to physical activity engagement?

And what if we learned how to recognize what we miss by looking for what we are likely not going to find?

Instead of considering activity participation narrowly, only as formal exercise (with accompanying resentment), how about considering engagement from the multi-dimensional enterprise that is physical activity and crediting ourselves for *all* the physical activity we have accrued? Instead of narrowly focusing upon the appearance transformation that isn't occurring, how about assessing the gain that *is* occurring? How about focusing on our accomplishments by acknowledging the benefits realized each time we engage in physical activity? How about broadly considering indices of physical activity success, and then showcasing our achievement?

And how about being excited about tomorrow's physical activity even while doing today's?

Welcome to Iron Footprint Fitness

Iron Footprint Fitness is an innovative approach to physical activity that fosters resilient motivation to sustain regular activity by reframing how engagement can be conceived and illustrating how achievement can be recognized. The realm of physical activity is an enterprise that is made up of multiple dimensions of engagement: health-related activity, activity separate or in addition to health-related activity, and performance benchmarks, and each dimension carries its unique indices of achievement. *Iron Footprint* is a graphic representation of our collective physical activity experience, our physical activity portfolio, which displays an account of our engagement and achievement as it occurs across the enterprise dimensions. Attributes of resiliency; hope, and autonomy are stoked upon 'seeing' the achievement we have rendered.

First, why *iron* footprint? What does *iron* have to do with sustaining resilient motivation to engage in regular physical activity?

The earliest pieces of equipment to aid physique development were made of iron, and most of today's equipment is still fabricated from some iron amalgam. Among barbells, dumbbells, or other manufactured free weights or lines of machines, the common material is iron, or a compounded derivative of the same. *Iron* is what is lifted, hoisted, pushed, pulled, pressed, and carried toward developing our physical selves. *Iron* also represents the equipment and action to engage our cardiovascular system. Most gym equipment that elicits a cardiovascular response—treadmills, ellipticals, stationary bikes, rowers, stair mills, and so on—appear to the naked eye to have at least a bit of iron in the machinery. Of the action itself that invokes our cardiovascular system (e.g., walking, running, swimming, cycling), just as iron is a critical building block used in construction (think rebar), cardio exercise is the primary building block of our health-related well-being.

Through history and still relevant today, *iron* is synonymous with the gym experience. It also represents physical activity outside the gym. From Merriam-Webster, *iron* is "a prospective course of action." Using creative license to assume prospective results in action, iron stands for all the games, activities, and experiences we have as we express our physical activity selves. Whether it is league softball, pick-up basketball, sea kayaking, rounds of golf, or sets of tennis, each is a course of action in which we have chosen to engage. Barring complications, while some physical activity is good, more is better. The more (physical activity) *irons* in the fire, the better.

Iron also captures the qualitative essence of physical activity achievement. From Merriam-Webster, *iron* connotes "strength, hardness, and determination." Ironman competitions are aptly named, considering these descriptors. Completing a two-mile swim, 112-mile bike ride, and 26.2 mile run for a single event is an ultimate test of physical aptitude. But any physical activity achievement requires the same qualities. Our physical activity portfolio, our *Iron Footprint*, will not be imprinted without purposeful and consistent effort. This requires the determination that characterizes *iron.*

Second, I sense your apprehension. I get that you have tried to try, and that you continue to try to try. I get that you have spent money in the effort to try to try. I get that you have gotten your hopes up that each new thing is the thing that will stick, the thing that will help you be motivated to do activity, only to be disappointed—again. So, I get that you *want* to think this could work for you but wonder if this is only "Here I go again."

I get that you also may feel like you have such an insignificant Iron Footprint that you doubt you even qualify to consider this approach to engagement and achievement. To that, I say yes, even you possess an Iron Footprint, for each of us is born with an innate impulse to *move*, as it's through movement that we learn about ourselves and our world. Through this process, we also impress our physical activity footprint, our *Iron Footprint*—a portfolio of our collected physical activity that begins at birth. Your Iron Footprint is as unique to you as mine is to me. It is also indelible and dynamic; its content can never be erased, and it is further impressed with each physical activity experience we accrue.

To that end, while it's easy to say we should let go of the past, it's our past that influences our future when it comes to physical activity participation, mainly for the way in which we have learned to approach engagement and regard achievement. While the motivation may ebb more than flow, and it may be due to less-than-optimal reasons, you do get to the gym or go for a run or walk because you seek body transformation. Yes, you know it's good for you, but body transformation drives participation and gauges success because other means for accomplishing those goals are not considered.

The narrower the target, though, the more likely a miss, and in this case you don't have more pitches to swing at. What results is the erosion of your motivation to sustain engagement. No choice here; we have to get past the past.

So what about *all* of the physical activity you do? What about *how* you do it? And what about the consistent engagement that you *do* manage to sustain?

Think about all the miles, repetitions, sets, revolutions, classes taken, push/pulls, laps, loops, intervals, or repeats you have done through the years. And consider this not just from the checkmark perspective ("Yes, I did it"), but also from a "Some days I felt really good and went faster than usual" perspective. Also think about all the tennis or pick-up basketball games played, golf rounds completed, swings taken at the batting cage, waves ridden, walks with your dog, or new fitness classes taken. As well, consider your participation habit itself. Even when having those 'just' days of self-negotiated light cardio exercise or weight training, in fact those were sessions of participation that deserve recognition with the "Yes, I did it" checkmark, especially considering the alternative of ending up on the couch at home rather than on an exercise bike at the gym.

What can this signify? What does this add up to—the *all* that you have done, the *how* it has been done, and the participation habit you *do* manage to sustain? What are you missing about your own physical activity achievement in the *all, how,* and *do* by narrowly focusing on one aspect of achievement that is unlikely to be realized, at least in the way it has been promised?

Physical activity is a *multi-dimensional enterprise* whose participation achievements can be framed and acknowledged in multiple ways. Iron Footprint Fitness offers the means to *broadly identify, capture and showcase physical activity achievement* so that *motivation* for further participation is *sustained*.

The Multi-Dimensional Enterprise That is Physical Activity and Physical Activity Participation

Physical activity is a multi-faceted enterprise of great depth and breadth, and participation brings with it wide-ranging impact. Running can clear the arteries and clear the head. Surfing can resonate with the synergy of the environment, along with the essence of our soul. Hitting a softball can evoke the thrill of contact. Trying a new group fitness class can produce adrenaline from anticipation.

All at once, it can be what we see, feel, sense, and smell. Viewing your engagement only along one dimension ("Yes, I did my cardio today" or "No, I didn't") doesn't nearly capture its magnitude. Nor does assessing your results only based upon body transformation ("My legs are still fat") access the innumerable ways that achievement within its engagement can be framed.

Do you remember the first time you saw color TV, high-def TV, 3-D TV? Or the first time you heard an orchestra? Or the first time you used the 32-color rather than the eight-color box of crayons?

Black and white TV projected an image, but the whole of the viewing experience changed with color, then high-def, then 3-D capability. Hearing the vocalization of a song can be pleasing, but hearing an orchestra project its tonal spectrum can evoke a profound emotional response. The eight-color box of crayons can suffice to draw a picture, but the 32-color box offers options for detail, precision, and clarity—the more from which self-expression can emerge.

So, too, regarding physical activity. Participation tends to be regarded like black and white TV, the vocalization of a song, or the eight-color box of crayons—comparatively primitive and superficial to how it *can* be considered. If we don't realize all we can from its engagement, motivation can erode, even for those who may not realize it is eroding.

Consider your relationships with music, literature, and food. Your relationship to music would likely change if, all of a sudden, you could only listen to one genre or one artist, neither being one you liked. Maybe you would listen for no reason other than to provide background noise, but your motivation to do so would not be nearly as strong as if you were able to listen to what you preferred. The same with literature and food. If you especially like poetry but were assigned science fiction, or wanted comic books but were given biographies, your motivation to read would drastically suffer. And eating the same thing day after day can provide basic sustenance, but would not generate excitement toward eating. And while salt and pepper are perfectly good flavor enhancers, how much more flavor would be possible with other types of seasoning?

Looking at it in a slightly different way, what if you only knew one genre of music or literature, or one type of food, not realizing others existed?

The realm of physical activity reaches far and wide—health-related exercise, team sports, individual sports, dance, martial arts, group fitness classes, aquatics, surfing, kayaking, yoga, leisurely bike rides. Each is a unique form of movement whose engagement can evoke different physical and emotional responses, and be the source from which to recount multi-varied achievement or success.

For example, on any given day you may complete your exercise routine—your workout—at a gym or outside of a gym. In addition, you may go for a walk, ride a bike, or play in your league softball game. Your workout may have been one where everything felt great and you outdid yourself, perhaps lifted more weight than ever, or reached 5,000 strides faster than ever on the elliptical machine. Or maybe it was a motivational struggle for you to complete your workout, but this one notched the most you have ever done in a row, and included taking part in the group fitness class you have had your eye on but hadn't yet been able to conjure the nerve to try.

Think about *all* the physical activity good you accomplished. You completed your workout *and* reached a new performance level *and* set your record for consistency *and* experienced a new activity *and* engaged in additional activity during the day. To recount the day's activity only according to "Yes, I did my workout today" sure does not come close to capturing its depth or significance. Taking stock of the day by looking at your legs in the mirror and declaring them "still fat" sure doesn't give credit where credit is due.

Physical activity participation is a multi-dimensional enterprise for which achievement is:

- Completing a health-related fitness workout.
- Engaging in activity separate from, and/or in addition to, a health-related workout.
- Trying a new activity.
- Setting a personal performance benchmark.

Makes sense!

But wait, I suck at sports, I dread doing my workout, I don't have the nerve to try new activities, I have two left feet when it comes to dance, I can't balance to stay on a surfboard, I'm too stiff to do yoga, I can't lift heavy weights, I'm a slow runner, I've never won an award in anything related to physical activity ...

Ahh, let the transformation begin. First things first though, before we can begin to assess achievement that reflects participation's multi-dimensional enterprise. We have to get beyond the negative perceived absolutes we carry about our relationship to physical activity.

Perceived Absolutes about Physical Activity: For Most of Us, Very Dangerous, Polarized Perceptions

It's no wonder we develop a one-dimensional, narrow perspective from which to consider the realm of physical activity, our engagement, and how to assess our achievement: we tend to form polarized absolutes in childhood that brand our physical activity identity and influence our lifelong participation tendencies.

Early, on the playground, we learn that games are either won or lost, and we either contribute or not to winning, or get blamed or not for losing. Even attempts to play without keeping score are thinly veiled efforts overshadowed by the final score and our contribution to that score. Related, there are no secrets when it comes to the playground pecking order. Our contribution, or lack thereof, to game success, determines the playground hierarchy, and mitigates team selection.

We either are excitedly chosen for a team or bear the humiliation of being added reluctantly.

We also learn early that physical fitness is either passed or failed, and unfortunately for most, the latter more than the former, with little recognition of improvement. Consider the pull-up test many of us did in elementary school. The test was either passed by completing requisite repetitions of pulling one's chin over the bar, or profoundly failed. Nor was there acknowledgment of post-test improvement, even if our pull increased from no attempt to *nearly* chin-over-bar.

Further, we learn early on that taking sides can be inherent to the physical activity experience, and toward which there are 'good guys' and 'bad guys.' There are the home team and the visiting team, the favorite and the underdog, the team we love and the team we love to hate. The strength of choice should never be underestimated, as often the sentiment toward the sides we choose only deepens as we grow older.

Early on, and in large part influenced by what occurs in that complex social arena that is the schoolyard playground, polarized absolutes about our relationship to physical activity take shape and form our physical activity identity.
We either:

- Succeed at physical activity *or* fail at physical activity.
- Are good at sports *or* are bad at sports.
- Like physical activity *or* dislike physical activity.
- Are active *or* are not active.

Fast forward to adulthood, and our consideration of physical activity remains aligned to the polarized identity that took shape during our formative years, except that now our conception of participation carries its own absolute and is even more narrowly considered:

- I play sports *or* I don't play sports.
- I like to exercise *or* I hate to exercise.
- I accept my body *or* I hate my body.
- I am an active person *or* I am not an active person.
- I protect my activity time *or* I make excuses to not be active.

- I seek optimal physical wellness *or* I seek the minimum recommended amount of exercise only because I know I should.
- I engage in physical activity for optimal physical wellness *or* I exercise to transform my body.

What is developed is a utilitarian, one-dimensional perspective through which we regard *exercise* as the entire realm of physical activity participation—the only form of physical activity in which we engage. Based upon our identity formed from past experience, we have written other forms off as impossible to consider, much less realistic to attempt.

In and of themselves, these adult absolutes don't necessarily have to play out as a negative. If we manage to sustain a regular, health-related fitness exercise routine, then we likely are able to realize health protective benefits. But what *is* dangerous is to judge our (fledgling) participation from the one-dimensional perspective carried from our early years, to assess physical activity as either winning or losing, especially insofar as this assessment is applied to the outcome most sought—body transformation.

With maturity, it seems that the polarity of winning and losing is tempered, or so we think. But sadly, because we don't know any differently, we consider ourselves to either win or lose at physical activity participation, defeat or be defeated. Combine this perspective with how millions of people frame achievement/success—magazine cover abs, arms like (insert celebrity/public figure here), legs like (insert celebrity/public figure here). A scenario is created in which realized outcomes are unlikely because the goals themselves are unrealistic.

Success or achievement, as we have come to define it, is nearly impossible to realize, and we miss the forest (indicators of health-related fitness) for the trees (body transformation), as achieving the trees we desire is fundamentally impossible to begin with. To add, while some transformation is certainly possible through exercise, it is all the more unlikely to occur if engagement is approached from a 'just' perspective, without consideration for the effort intensity required to induce any transformation.

Whew!

And so it is that we set ourselves up for failure and, ultimately, for quitting exercise, the only form of physical activity in which we engage to begin with.

Why?

Because the polarized absolutes—and the resulting narrow, one-dimensional perspective from which we consider physical activity engagement and judge achievement, *can erode motivation.*

Pulsing along a spectrum, motivation drives behavior and determines if and how physical activity is engaged. Absolutes formed early can profoundly influence lifelong physical activity participation patterns, especially considering how they impact aspects of resiliency: hope and autonomy.

If you generalize along the positives, your motivation to engage in physical activity likely has been steadfast. You probably possess a dense accumulation of broad-based experiences that you have unabashedly conveyed along the way. Occurrences at games and practices are conversation topics for as long as they make a good story. The gym is the same. The sets and reps 'nailed' or the cardio exercise 'cranked out.' Not to suggest that this reflects boorish form, rather it is healthy self-reporting slanted toward a sense of achievement or success. You likely possess a strong sense of who you are related to physical activity. Not to imply that you are an elite athlete who has competed on the world stage, but rather that your physical activity personality is aptly developed so as to feel pride about this piece of your identity. Importantly, you are confidently optimistic that your forthcoming activity engagement will be positive, affirming, and meaningful.

Sadly, for many, engagement is anything but. Untold millions generalize otherwise, and their motivation to engage suffers. Two-thirds of all American adults carry unhealthy weight, and approximately 60 million are clinically obese. Over one-quarter fail to accumulate **any** leisure time physical activity. Compared to those who skew along positive absolutes, accounts of experiences dredge up humiliation and failure, without any resonance. The accumulation of total activity is thin, as engagement is dreaded to the point of avoidance. What comes first? Avoidance, lack of perceived success, or a thin activity portfolio? Hard to say, other than physical activity autonomy is wholly underdeveloped, if even a blip on the radar. We essentially become adversaries to our physical selves. We are disconnected to our bodies and feel contempt for perceived incompetence. And hope for anything different is nonexistent. Optimism that our future activity experience will be positive, or that we can realize success? Please! And now I'm supposed to go to the gym to do what? And for how long? Right. "I'm bad at sports, therefore I will never be able to achieve at sports, therefore there is nothing for me to consider as achievement" or "My legs are still fat so I'm not successful at exercise." Exercise wins, I lose!

The effort to participate becomes second to the effort required to become motivated to participate. It can be draining—the push/pull. The "I know I should, but I'm not any good at it" struggle. "Why should I continue to try when I never see results?" Expectation of achievement is either dismissed or wholly given up on, but given the insidiously narrow, unrealistic perspective from which it has been considered, it was virtually impossible to begin with. After all, absolutes are absolutes! Achievement and success (winning) consist of only the magazine cover abs or arms or legs I develop, but will (likely) never develop, yet I will win only if this is achieved.

Ugh!

Not only does this approach subvert the whole of physical activity, it literally wagers health protection. And it helps explain why quieting the gremlins that start to chirp the moment we begin to contemplate going to the gym is more complicated than it may seem.

But wait—let's return to those early days on the playground. Remember what happened when it couldn't be determined if the ball was fair or foul? Or if the player was safe or out? Or when something unexpected caused some sort of interference? A do-over was declared, and the game reverted to the action point of the disputed incident.

Considering the tangled web that could be woven during playground games, could there be anything as useful and satisfying as the do-over? For upon its declaration, peace was instantly restored, dissonance forgotten, and the game began again with renewed zest and energy.

This is your do-over!

So, in the spirit of do-overs, it's time to:

- Recognize the realm of physical activity as a multi-dimensional enterprise.
- Approach your engagement from this multi-dimensional perspective.
- Broadly consider and frame achievement and success as they align to the process and products that emerge from considering engagement from this multi-dimensional perspective.

- Build resilient motivation to engage in physical activity by accessing success.

The really good news is that this is a simple and wholly painless modification to your approach and account of physical activity that can be **IT** toward helping you reconnect (or further connect) and sustain your motivation to engage. Back to a few paragraphs ago—wouldn't it be a relief to ease your day-to-day struggle of summoning motivation to be active? And gratifying to realize the parallel achievement and success that you reap? Too, wouldn't it be satisfying to really know all you have accomplished in the realm of activity? And all without having to spend any money!

Using contemporary vernacular, physical activity is a 'blue sky' entity. There is virtually endless possibility as to what we can do in its name, then for how to recount achievement and success. Yet, we narrowly pigeon-hole what we allow ourselves to do and how we judge achievement. Yep, those darn absolutes again. But the past is the past, and it's 'blue sky' we have to look forward to as we rid ourselves of our absolutes that only hurt … ourselves. The do-over begins now. Back to Iron Footprint.

So how to access achievement within your Iron Footprint to foster resilient exercise motivation? Create an icon that showcases your engagement across its dimensions.

Your Iron Footprint is a portfolio of your collected physical activity according to how it occurs across the enterprise. It is graphically represented by an icon that illustrates your accumulation of health-related activity, activity engaged in separate from that which is health-related, all the different types of activity engaged in, and performance bench-marks. It is further imprinted upon each occurrence of physical activity participation.

If physical activity is engaged according to the protocol required to yield health-related benefit, results corresponding to measures of health protection are (relatively) likely. While many of us heed physical activity's 'good for us' virtue, and appreciate improved measures of wellness, this doesn't necessarily truthfully capture our participation motive—radical body transformation. Even with physical wellness improvement, engagement motivation can be undermined when we perceive that transformation is not occurring.

Hoped-for radical transformation is wholly unrealistic to begin with, but especially unfortunate when missing the significant gains that *are* made—that were never considered.

Imprinting your Iron Footprint shifts the focus from looking for what you don't perceive to be occurring (failure) to realizing what is occurring (successes) by illustrating the innumerable ways that success is realized. It counters the absolutes "I'm bad at sports" (so I'm not going to try) and "I hate to exercise" (because I've never felt successful) by providing a frame for articulating, and then depicting, achievement. It helps us to think differently about the knowing, the doing, and how to assess participation for both process and product outcomes.

We *know* we need to exercise for our health, but what do you really *know* about *you* and the physical activity enterprise?

- Do you know how many push ups you can do in one minute?
- Do you know how many days in a row you were able to do your workout?
- Do you know how many steps you can accumulate in 20 minutes on the elliptical?
- Do you know how far you can throw a softball?
- Do you know how many different activities you have tried?
- Do you know how long you can hold a plank?

You deserve to reap *all* the good that can be had from physical activity—health protection, fun, satisfaction, pride, confidence—and realize participation from positive absolutes. Accounting for the consistency with which you complete your health-related workout, crediting yourself for engaging in activity separate from your workout and taking in new activity experiences, and notching personal performance benchmarks deepens the meaning of physical activity participation by capturing indices of success from the multi-dimensions that comprise the enterprise.

Acknowledging participation ought to be much more complex than simply logging a session of requisite time and check-marking its completion. For during that time or experience, you may have achieved a personal best in some aspect of cardio exercise, strength training, or skill execution. Or you may have finally managed the nerve to take a group fitness class that has intrigued, yet intimidated, you. Success is completing your health-related workout, success is engaging in activity separate from your workout, success is adding a new activity to your profile, and success is setting a personal benchmark.

The purpose of creating your Iron Footprint icon is to showcase the multiple ways that you realize success in the realm of physical activity engagement. While this approach cannot guarantee achievement, it can guarantee *access* to your achievement. Also, while this approach can help to focus your activity engagement (as will be described further), it is not a prescriptive workout to follow, rather the complement to *any* prescriptive workout followed. For example, numerous commercial exercise programs exist to aid the development of fitness (e.g., Crossfit, 10 Minute Trainer, Total Gym, The Rack, The Jack Rack, Insanity, P90X). Any one of these programs could be suitable to follow in your quest for physical wellness. The point here is Iron Footprint Fitness is program neutral and program useful. Its purpose is to transform your conception of engagement and achievement in order to foster resilient motivation to sustain a regular activity habit. Iron Footprint Fitness is also personal trainer-neutral, meaning you can use it even if you work with a personal trainer. In fact, if a trainer dissuaded you from using it, I'd regard that as a red flag to switch to a different trainer.

• • •

Summary and a Peek Ahead

With that, we leave the past as an 'ago'. We have let go of the perceived absolutes that weigh so heavily on our effort to be active, chased the clouds away that darken how we feel about our physical selves, allowed ourselves to take a do-over, and learned how to forever quiet the gremlins. With our physical activity psyche now filled with—dare I say—optimism about engagement, what's that I hear knocking at the door? Well, it looks like, it smells like, yes, it's resilient motivation. Go ahead, open the door.

The next section describes Iron Footprint's parameters and offers the definitions for identifying, capturing and showcasing achievement for each dimension of engagement.

PART II

THE FEATURES AND CONTOURS OF THE ENGAGEMENT DIMENSIONS ACHIEVEMENT FOR EACH

Physical activity is a multi-dimensional enterprise whose engagement includes participation done as one's health-related workout, participation done separate from or in addition to one's health-related workout, and consideration for the quality of engagement. Achievement is recognized by accounting for:

- Each completed health-related fitness workout.
- Engagement that is separate from or in addition to one's workout, and all the different types of activities in which one has engaged.
- Personal performance benchmarks.

Counter to how its engagement is often considered and its outcomes often judged, physical activity is a multi-dimensional enterprise for which achievement can be considered in multiple ways. This relieves the dangerously narrow mindset that typically characterizes our approach to, and account of, our engagement—dangerous because of how it can erode our motivation to sustain a regular activity habit. Iron Footprint Fitness is a transformed approach to physical activity engagement that renovates our consideration and regard for success.

Part II matches concept to application. Each dimension of the Iron Footprint physical activity enterprise is described for its unique features and contours, and for how achievement can be considered. The purpose of Part II is to stoke the creation of your Iron Footprint icon.

Your Health-Related Physical Activity Habit—Your Exercise Workout

Physical activity is commonly engaged as one's workout routine, or activity focused upon fostering health-related fitness. This is what we do toward the sentiment of 'exercising because we know it's good for us.' For the best reason, sustaining a health-related workout habit is a vital backbone to our physical and emotional well-being.

This type of participation ought to occur daily, or as close to daily as possible, and with intensity appropriate to induce health protection. Physical vigor and vitality cannot be banked, so this type of physical activity engagement isn't to be negotiated, especially if the negotiation is to leverage future days off. Nor should this type of engagement be rationed (considerations for safety notwithstanding). We know what we need to do toward fostering cardiovascular, muscular, and joint fitness, and need to engage accordingly. This dimension of engagement fosters healthy (or healthier) markers of wellness.

(*Note* – a description of the protocol required to stimulate health-related benefit from engagement is outlined in *Achievement-Oriented Health-Related Fitness: What We Need to Know* located in Part IV of this book and as a download at www.ironfootprintfitness.com.)

Achievement in this dimension is acknowledged by recognizing your consistency. Since this type of engagement most directly focuses upon fostering and protecting our physical well-being, credit is to be notched for each workout you complete where you have engaged according to the principles required to impact health-related fitness. The ongoing accumulation of notches represents the crucial health-protective aspect of consistency. This is success!

The Physical Activity You Do Separate from Your Daily Workout, and, All the Different Types of Physical Activity in Which You Have Participated

Physical activity engagement often occurs separate from, or in addition to, activity that comprises your daily workout. For example, on any given day, either before or after your workout, you might also go for a bike ride, play pick-up basketball, or take a yoga class. This type of activity tends to be characterized differently from activity engaged in for a workout and represents a different dimension of movement, approached more from the perspective of fun ("Yippee, I get to go on a bike ride") than as an obligation (not that workouts ought to be dreaded, but you get the point). Related, the intensity of engagement tends to be more moderate than vigorous, and its focus is more on the experience of the activity itself rather than on how it will foster components of health-related fitness (e.g., cardiovascular or muscular strength). There is an obvious categorical difference in purpose and intent between, say, surfing and lifting weights at the gym.

As with a comparison among chocolate, vanilla, and strawberry ice cream, the point is not to rank order. While each is a cold, creamy treat, each carries a distinct flavor that brands its uniqueness. This dimension of the physical activity enterprise encompasses and accounts for all the different types of activities that are engaged. To be clear, this is not to suggest that one ought to forego engagement in one dimension (weight-lifting) for engagement in another (surfing). In general, you can't reap from surfing what you can reap from weight-lifting, and vice-versa.

Acknowledging achievement in this dimension involves notching *all* the physical activity you do separate from, or in addition to, your workout, and notching each new activity you try. Some activity participation is good, but more is better, so it is an achievement when you engage in activity apart from your workout. It's also an achievement when you engage in a new activity, since doing so requires that a certain degree of risk has been overcome.

The Quality of Your Engagement—How You Engage

Engagement in physical activity lends itself to tracking measures of performance. What is the fastest ever run? Farthest ever thrown? Highest ever jumped? Most weight ever lifted? Encompassing a multitude of different forms of movement, each of these is a metric that represents the third dimension of the physical activity enterprise—the quality of engagement, or *how* you have engaged.

Acknowledging achievement in this dimension entails noting your personal records or performance benchmarks. Elite athletes are routinely scrutinized according to their performance statistics. Considering how media growth has increased the number of platforms that provide analysis and how technology has enhanced the detail that is analyzed, multi-varied evaluation occurs instantaneously. Cumulatively, statistics profile performance capacity and represent the wonderment of the physical bounds of human achievement. Just how fast, far, high can we go?

But, you might think, I'm not a professional or elite athlete—heck, compared to others I see on the treadmill at the gym, I'm not even in their league. So why does it matter that I track my performance benchmarks? Why should I keep my own statistics?

Personal bests are personal bests. Whether a world record set at the Olympic Games or a personal benchmark set at the local gym, the meaning is the same. It signifies success in the form of performance improvement, which is a source of pride and satisfaction, and feeds motivation. Tracking benchmarks opens innumerable opportunities for success to be captured. It counters the narrow perspective from which success tends to be considered—the absolute of winning or losing determined only by body transformation. Rather, success is realized by recognizing improvement. Maybe you are not yet able to complete a full pull-up, but now you can pull to the top of your head after being barely able to sustain an elbow bend last week. Or now you are able to walk one mile on the treadmill in 15 minutes after clocking 17 minutes last week. This is success; it is achievement and ought to be recognized as such.

The beauty in tracking physical activity performance measures is the fact that there are virtually infinite opportunities to do so. And, because your body is the only one you've got, you ought to develop your physical self as fully as possible. This means striving to set personal bests and compiling your performance statistics. World records? Probably not. Recognition from others? Probably not (unless you share your good fortune). But you will notice your pride and self-confidence blossoming as you witness yourself improving, getting stronger and faster, going farther and longer.

To recap this section, noting consistency, accounting for all the activity you accrue, and tracking performance measures transform your assessment of your physical activity experience beyond the hollow absolutes of "Yes, I was active today" or "No, I wasn't active today," recounting simply time or distance logged, and considering success only for body transformation. Recognizing achievement as it occurs across the dimensions of the enterprise adds substance and meaning to the experience, and most importantly, nourishes resilient motivation. Achievement begets achievement! Success begets success! Hope and autonomy spring forth and feed your motivation for continued engagement.

•   •   •

Translating the Features and Contours of the Engagement Dimensions into Your Iron Footprint Icon--SEE Your Achievement

Your Iron Footprint is a portfolio of your collective physical activity experience. It is comprised of accounts of engagement that occur across the dimensions that make up the enterprise of physical activity. Achievement respective to each dimension is showcased by creating an Iron Footprint icon, a graphic depiction of your physical activity portfolio.

> *Your Iron Footprint **showcases** your physical activity **achievement** as a portfolio of **FitBASE**-daily fitness routine, **FitBUBBLES**- accumulation of physical activity and **FitBESTS**-performance benchmarks. The tangible display of your physical activity self and your achievement has a powerful influence on your motivation to sustain regular activity. Success begets success! Approaching physical activity as Iron Footprint Fitness can motivate you to engage every day.*

Now comes the fun part – creating your Iron Footprint to showcase your portfolio of physical activity achievement. The following explains how to translate your collective physical activity experience into your Iron Footprint according to the features and contours of the FitBASE, FitBEST and FitBUBBLES dimensions.

FitBASE Dimension: *Your Achievement-Oriented Health-Related Fitness Routine (Your Workout)*

This dimension of activity is what you do specifically to impact your health-related wellness. This is "I do it because it's good for me" engagement, also commonly referred to as exercise, or one's routine or workout.

Considering the profound influence that this dimension of activity has on our well-being its engagement ought to be consistent, optimally daily, and because its impact is so profound, this dimension bears strong labeling—It *is* the BASE upon which quality of life depends by providing the foundation of physical wellness.

FitBASE achievement is completing an achievement-oriented health-related workout (AOHR). Notching your Iron Footprint with each completed workout will result in an ever –growing line or sequence of marks. Since consistency of engagement in this dimension of activity is of foremost importance, displaying your accumulated pattern shows clear evidence that you *have* stuck to a routine. Seeing your strings of consecutive days of engagement provides impetus to sustain your pattern.

To imprint your FitBASE:

Decide a scheme for how you want to recognize each AOHR workout that you complete at the gym or otherwise (e.g., running or walking outside for cardiovascular benefit rather than using a cardio machine at the gym). For example, you can use a weekly or monthly calendar to X off each day you complete an AOHR workout, or you can color in sections of a pillar shape until the pillar is filled in and you begin to color in a new pillar (vertical recognition), or add a notch to an ongoing arrow (horizontal recognition). Use the available tools on 'My Iron Footprint' to style this dimension of your Iron Footprint.

For engagement to qualify for FitBASE notation it must include activity of each health-related fitness component (cardiovascular strength, muscular strength and endurance, flexibility) and adhere to each component's achievement principles:

- Cardiovascular strength: 30 minutes minimum of aerobic exercise with your heart rate sustained in your training zone.
- Muscular strength or mass: Weight training to build strength or mass.
- Flexibility: Stretching for the purpose of increasing joint range-of-motion using a mix of static and dynamic movement, or completing a pilates, yoga, or similar session.

(*Note* – please refer to *Achievement-Oriented Health-Related Fitness: What We Need to Know* in the Iron Footprint Fitness Academy Library White Paper downloads at ironfootprintfitness.com for a description of the protocol required to stimulate health-related benefit from engagement.)

FitBUBBLE Dimension: *1) Activity Done In Addition To Or Separate From Your Workout, And 2) Each Different Physical Activity You Have Tried*

For reasons that tend to differ from those that inspire our FitBASE workout, we also engage in activity that is separate from or in addition to our workout. Perhaps called 'leisure' or 'recreational', this dimension of activity participation is typically engaged less intensely than FitBASE, and for reasons more varied. For example, on a day where we have already notched our FitBASE workout, we may also take an evening bike ride to prepare for a triathlon, play a league softball game to feed our sense of competition or invite someone to go for a walk to reconnect.

This dimension of activity represents another aspect of our activity profile as it is another way we express our physical self compared to our FitBASE. Each of these occurrences is captured for your Iron Footprint as a FitBUBBLE. A FitBUBBLE is an activity that is done *separate from or in addition to* your daily FitBASE. *Each different type* of physical activity in which you have engaged also merits a FitBUBBLE.

Until you write it down, you may not realize all the different types of physical activity you have tried. Sports, aquatics, forms of dance, fitness classes; the list can go on and on. While it may not be an infinite list, it's definitely extensive. So, too, is how the source of participation can be considered, be it in organized or informal instances, occurring inside or outside the gym, during physical education class or on your own.

FitBUBBLES display all the different forms of physical activity that you have tried, and credits the positive lifestyle choice of engaging in activity beyond your requisite daily workout. Beyond reasons related to health protection, participating in physical activity is simply a good way to spend time. Chunking FitBUBBLES will give you the impetus to continue participating in physical activity in addition to your daily workout and to keep trying new activities. 'Collecting' activity and trying new activities is achievement, creates new opportunities to realize achievement and success, and further develops your physical activity personality.

Initially, this dimension of your portfolio may be comparatively underdeveloped because you have never considered accounting for participation in this way. Perhaps you haven't purposefully tried nor had the opportunity to try a wide variety of different physical activities. Or maybe you lack confidence to try new activities stemming from a fixed absolute—"I fail at physical activity, therefore I am not going to try anything new!" Trying a new activity can be risky, especially with a history of perceived failure. It can take gumption to stir the nerve to engage beyond your perceived limits. Achievement is in taking the risk.

You may be content with doing your 'regular' activity either inside or outside the gym, e.g., attending the same group fitness class or jogging the same three-mile course. Participating solely in one type of physical activity can yield important health-protective outcomes—a densely developed repertoire of activity isn't needed to realize benefit—but a critical aspect of reaping full benefit from the physical activity enterprise is to develop your physical activity personality by seeking to experience all physical activity, then acknowledging and revering each new experience.

Otherwise, *your* physical activity self can be left to others to dictate, and limited options mean just that—limited options. Not to mention that this brings you right back to feeling 'assigned' to do something, which increases the chances we will rebel against it. While participating in a group fitness class can result in critical health-related benefit, *your* physical activity self will be developed according to the instructor's perspective, and that form of activity may not evoke all *your* senses.

The 'same' becomes too routine when it stunts motivation, and a portfolio that is thin, with only a few different activity experiences included, prompts underachievement, as it lessens the opportunities for success. Along with trying new experiences come infinite possibilities for achievement and success. For example, as is presented in the next section, FitBESTS are personal records for broadly considered activity events. The more activities in which you participate the more opportunity you create to set (and reset) personal records. Achievement recognition exponentially increases the deeper your portfolio. FitBUBBLES acknowledge the participation itself while FitBESTS acknowledge the quality of the participation.

Your Iron Footprint FitBUBBLES ought to become dense and clustered as you begin to realize and experience the multiple ways you can grow this aspect of your physical activity portfolio. You want your

FitBUBBLE display to seem like its buzzing! as the act of collecting things can be self-generating—the more we collect, the more we want to collect. It can also foster respect for what is collected and be a source of celebration when more is added. Considering how physical activity participation can positively impact your quality of life, collecting physical activity is a good thing to collect!

Ultimately, the more developed your physical activity personality, the more likely it is that your motivation to sustain a regular activity habit will be stable.

(Note: The antithesis of healthy collecting is developing an obsession where other facets of life are neglected. Like any addiction, an addiction to exercise can be devastating. This dimension of activity engagement is encouraged for the positive impact it can foster on your quality of life. Its inclusion is not meant to be cavalier to anyone who contends with addiction.)

To imprint FitBUBBLES:

Notch (as its own FitBUBBLE) each physical activity that you have ever tried *and* the physical activity done separate or in addition to your daily routine.

I.   What are *all* the *different* physical activities that you have ever tried? Consider:

- Team sports
- Individual sports
- Combatives
- Aesthetic activities
- Racquet sports
- Aquatic activities
- Leisure pursuits, e.g., bowling
- Group fitness classes

Even if you tried an activity only once, notch each different activity as its own FitBUBBLE. Add to your FitBUBBLE cluster by continuing to engage in activity that is novel to you. For example, take a golf or tennis lesson, rock climb, take a new group fitness or dance class, take a paddleboard lesson, learn to snowshoe. Each new activity you engage in enriches your physical activity profile and deepens your physical activity personality.

II.   What physical activity did you do *separate* or *in addition to* your daily routine? Consider:

- Motor skill practice.
- Sports league games or practices, or pick-up games.
- Organized road events—running, cycling, walking, mud/obstacle races.
- Cardio-related, but cardio-lite, activity (low intensity that is different, and in addition to, what was done for your daily cardiovascular workout (e.g., walking, biking, rollerblading, swimming, dancing).
- Skill-based leisure (low intensity) activity (e.g., golfing, bowling, surfing, skiing,skating, snowboarding, canoeing/kayaking, batting cage or driving range).

Add a FitBUBBLE to your cluster each time you engage in physical activity separate from or in addition to your daily workout. Since some physical activity is good, but more is better, the 'more' that we do deserves recognition. Considering the choices we have for how to spend leisure time, it is a lifestyle success to choose physical activity engagement.

Under-developed motor skills prevent participating in physical activities that require a certain proficiency. For example, if you are not able to competently dribble a basketball or throw a football or hit a forehand shot it is highly unlikely that you will seek to play basketball, football or tennis. Under-developed motor skills limit engagement opportunity [and how we regard our physical self], but proficiency CAN be developed through practice. For this reason, Iron Footprint Fitness includes motor skill practice as a component of an engagement routine. Please see *Add Motor Skill Practice To Your Routine—Why?* in the Iron Footprint Fitness Academy Library White Paper downloads for information about motor skills and a description of how to include their practice into your routine.)

FitBUBBLE Ideas/Resources

Even if you are motivated to do so, participating in activities that are new to you may be a challenge due to a variety reasons including financial constraints, geography, and accessible facilities. Consider the following resources for opportunities to add new activities to your FitBUBBLE cluster:

- Community college activity courses
- City/county recreation centers/community centers
- One-week or one-day passes to different gyms
- Community-based physical activity clubs, e.g., 'active singles' clubs. Look for ads in newspapers and on the internet.
- Physical education classes at K-12 schools – volunteer to assist the physical education teacher
- Batting cages and golf driving ranges – each offers an inexpensive way to experience baseball/softball batting and golf. Each also usually has equipment available for those who need it.

FitBEST Dimension: *Your Physical Activity Performance Benchmarks (Personal Best Records)*

What are your physical activity personal BESTS?

How fast can you run? How high can you jump? How far can you throw? Considering BESTS more broadly, how many push-ups can you do? How many steps can you accrue on the elliptical machine in 10 minutes? How long can you hold a plank pose?

Your physical activity portfolio, your Iron Footprint, is an accounting of the consistency in which you engage (FitBASE) and your accumulation of activity (FitBUBBLES). A third dimension of participation to recognize is accounting for *how* participation is completed. It goes without saying, but physical activity can inherently lead to the tracking of performance measures, especially for comparisons between people. Whose mark is the fastest? Highest? Strongest? Farthest? While on the world stage, the quest for 'est' can inspire unprecedented feats of physical achievement, the quest for your 'ests' is equally as important.

Your 'ests' are your physical activity performance benchmarks, or your personal FitBESTS.

A FitBEST is your personal record in a specific physical activity. It is important to clarify that the intent is not to assess your measures in comparison to anyone else's. Rather, noting your benchmarks is the means to track *your own* progress vis-à-vis a broadly-considered menu of physical activity 'events.' Tracking benchmarks displays tangible evidence of the gains (improvement) you are making. This overtly showcases the achievement (success) you garner. Compiling benchmarks, collecting 'ests', confirms the development of your physical self. Net/net, your very vim, vigor, and vitality emerge in front of your eyes.

To imprint FitBESTS:

First, brainstorm to compile a list of your physical activity performance benchmarks to date. If you have competed in organized sports or organized physical activity events (e.g., road races), this is a good place to start, especially if your engagement includes events of a defined distance (e.g., 5K run, 10K run) that are measured by time. Compare your finishing times (if you recorded them) and note your bests for the distances you have completed. Each separate best time and distance for which you have a measure is a FitBEST to be notched as part of your Iron Footprint.

But further, while notching organized sports or physical activity events measures provides a natural starting point, Iron Fitness Footprint benchmarks should be considered generously, and not just for how they occur in 'traditional,' sanctioned events.

FitBESTS should then be organized according to the innumerable ways that achievement can be measured within the cardiovascular, strength training, and motor skill-related aspects of your routine, or what you do outside your routine. Each benchmark is an achievement entitled to recognition and celebration. Recognition of accomplishment is not only for elite or professional athletes whose extraordinary feats result in world records or world championships. Personal records are as meaningful to you and me as world records are to them.

*FitBEST Event Trials Bank

The following are events that you can try as FitBEST trials. The bank includes those that you can do at the gym and/or at home, and those that occur as organized, community-based competitions.

*SAFETY is especially important when you attempt FitBESTS. This includes, but is not limited to: being healthy enough to attempt events that require intense exertion, using a qualified spotter, being proficient in the movement (using correct weight lifting techniques and using supports if needed, e.g., weight belts, knee/wrist straps), ensuring a debris-free area, etc.

Also:

- Be consistent in how you perform events from one trial of the same event to the next
- Wait at least 2 weeks before repeating an attempt
- Avoid using extra motion cheats (e.g., kipping during pull-ups)

Note – FitBESTS: A 14-Day Start-Up Plan presents how to begin to include attempts into your routine and *30-Days of 'BESTS* presents an extended plan. The former is included in Part IV of this book and both are available as White Papers of the Iron Footprint Fitness Academy on ironfootprintfitness.com.

Muscular Strength

- 1-Repetition Maximum (RM) lifts for bench press, bicep curl, squat, dead lift, overhead press – can be done using machines or free weights

Muscular Endurance

- Total repetitions of a specific weight of a specific exercise – e.g., bench press, bicep curl, squat, dead lift, overhead press, lat pulldown, tricep extension, hamstring curl, etc. These can be done using machines or free weights (barbells and/or dumb-bells) and at different angels of each exercise, where appropriate (inclines, declines, etc.)

- Bench press repetitions of body weight or 50% of body weight – this is often considered a signature exercise so is included separately from the above event idea
- Push-ups (modified or regular starting position): total, in one minute, total at an incline, total at a decline, total with hands forming a diamond
- Sit-ups / Abdominals: total (at flat and incline positions), in one minute (at flat and incline positions), holding a plank for as long as possible, holding a one-legged plank as long as possible
- Dips – total either assisted or unassisted, with or without added weight
- Pull-ups (palms facing away from body) / Chin-ups (palms facing toward body): total full-extension repetitions, total partial-extension repetitions (elbows bent to 45 degrees), total repetitions pulling to the top of your head, flexed arm hang hold for time. These can be assisted (using spotter or machine) or unassisted. If assisted, the trials can be conducted according to how many plates you use to assist your effort
- Holding 5lb, 10lb, 25lb, etc., weight plates in front of body for time. Maintain the position of looking through the center hole of the weight plate to ensure it stays in a fixed spot.
- Hold a tripod pose for time

Cardiovascular Capacity
At gym using cardiovascular machines:

- Steps completed in X minutes on the elliptical (at X level, at X incline)
- Time to get to 10,000 steps on the elliptical machine
- Time to 1 mile, 2 miles, 3 miles, etc., on the treadmill, stationary bike, rowing machine (at X level or incline)
- 1-mile repeat walks/runs hitting a specific time with an established rest interval – i.e., how many times can you walk 1-mile under 12 minutes with 2 minutes rest in-between each attempt?
- (X distance repeats of walking, running, cycling, elliptical, rowing, etc. hitting a specific time with an established rest interval)

- Time for gym triathlon: 1-mile on treadmill + 1-mile on stationary bike + 1-mile on elliptical (or X steps)

Outside of the gym (occurring as unorganized trials or during organized competitions/events):

- 1M, 5K, 10K, half-marathon, marathon walk, run, cycle, rollerblade
- Split times that occur during the above trials – e.g., 1-mile splits during a 5K or 10K run, half-marathon split during a full marathon, last mile of any event
- Furthest distance walked, run, cycled, rollerbladed

Miscellaneous cardiovascular-related engagement:

- 500, 1000 yard, mile swim (1650 yards)
- Jumping Rope – consecutive jumps, time to 100, 500, etc., jumps, using different skipping variations (see exercise tips for examples of different skipping styles)
- Step-Ups – using a 6" or 12" step, and either weighted (holding a weight) or non-weighted – total steps in 1-minute, 5-minutes, 20-minutes; time it takes to reach 100 total steps; alternating steps

Home Exercise Trials

- Landmark walking, running, cycling, rollerblading – establish a fixed distance – e.g., around the block, from one street sign to the next street sign, from one store front to another store front – how many times around the block in X minutes, fastest time around the block,
- Stairwell Step-Ups – total steps in 1-minute, 20-minutes; time it takes to reach 100 total steps; weighted (holding hand weights) or non-weighted
- Playground Facility Trials – mixed event obstacle course (under, over, across, around, through obstacles), monkey bar cross for time and endurance, pull-ups using a cross bar

Flexibility

- Hamstring measure - Sit-and-Reach distance, from standing position touch toes/knuckles/palms/forearms.
- Shoulder measure - Reaching down across your back (single arms), touching fingertips (one arm reaching down across your neck while the other reaches up around your back)
- Leg splits

Motor Skills / Sport-Related Performance Events

- Softball/baseball throw for distance
- Football punt/kick for distance
- Soccer punt/kick for distance
- Juggling two or three tennis balls for time
- Agility/Shuttle run – set out two cones (or suitable markers) approximately 20 feet apart. Begin at one cone, run around the second cone and back as quickly as possible. Variations: set four cones in a square formation approximately 20 feet from each other. Begin at one corner and running to the right circle the first cone, then the second, then the third, until finishing at the first cone; set 10 cones/markers an equal distance apart in a straight line of approximately 50 feet. Zig-zag around the cones (as if slalom skiing) from one end and back again; set four cones in a diamond pattern approximately 20 feet from each other. Begin at one cone and facing in shuffle to the first cone, then face out and shuffle to the second cone, then face in and shuffle to the third cone, then face out and shuffle to the beginning cone
- Standing Broad Jump
- Vertical Jump
- Platform Jump – successfully jumping onto a platform of X height
- 50, 100, 200, 400, 800 yard/meter dash

Combinations (events that combine elements of muscular and cardio-vascular capacity)

- Time to walk/run/cycle/row/elliptical X miles/steps on tread-mill/stationary bike/machine while doing 10 push-ups every 1-minute
- Super Set Circuit – time to complete 10 repetitions each of dumbbell bench press, bicep curl, overhead press, lat row, bench squats, tricep extension, and calf raises (this attempt requires access to varied dumbbell weights at once so may not be realistic for everyone)

  Note – CrossFit™ is a commercial exercise program that focuses on functional movement and movement combinations. Please access www.crossfit.com for more information about this type of an exercise program. Its approach is inherently complimentary to Iron Footprint Fitness.

Wellness Markers:
Blood pressure, resting heart rate, body composition, BMI, VO2max, cholesterol, blood sugar, bone density
> *Note* - Physical activity may not be the only variable that impacts wellness markers but experts agree about its contribution.

Examples of Sport-Specific FitBESTS:
Basketball
> Dribbling around obstacles for time
> Hot-shot spot shooting
> Passing accuracy: chest, bounce, overhead

Football
> 40yd dash
> Up/Downs
> Passing accuracy
> Receiving (catching): consecutive, building repertoire (catches to right/
left/above waist/below waist/over shoulder right/over shoulder left

More to Notch: Cognitive and Affective Indices of Engagement

Cognitive Aspects of Engagement

FitBASE, FitBUBBLES and FitBESTS capture achievement as it occurs across the dimensions of physical activity, but there is more about engagement that can be notched. Cognitive (knowledge) and affective (emotional) aspects of the physical activity experience also influence our motivation to participate, and in your quest to develop resilient motivation, this tracking adds additional acknowledgement to your portfolio.

Cognitive indices include how much content knowledge we possess—how much we know—about the realm of physical activity. Content knowledge related to physical activity includes understanding scientific principles of training, knowing rules and strategies to sports and games, and acquiring information as a fan of activity (e.g., accounts of others' engagement—both elite athletes and everyday gym-goers, and staying abreast of current sports events).

The greater your content knowledge, the more likely you will sustain engagement, for knowledge can impact motivation by inducing confidence, mitigating self-direction, increasing choice, and maintaining perspective. For example, if you are a 'student' of physical activity who understands the scientific principles of engagement, the more you will be assured that your engagement *will* yield results. The assurance is priceless, for you spend zero psychic energy wondering if what you are doing is right and hoping you are not wasting your time. Similarly, the more you know, the less you have to rely on anyone else to guide your activity, which means the greater self-direction you employ toward structuring your activity time. A caveat here for those of you who work with personal trainers. You likely do so with good reason. Trainers can be invaluable partners, but ultimately our engagement is ours to own. The more it is self-directed, the greater our motivation and likelihood that we will sustain regular engagement.

Enhanced content knowledge also triggers a deepened activity portfolio that allows for choice of engagement on any given day. This can mean engagement considered from the macro level, e.g., deciding between tennis or golf, and engagement considered from the micro level, e.g., deciding between free weights or weight machines. 'Choice' has a positive impact on engagement motivation. It affords variety, which maintains freshness, which translates to anticipation and optimism. This leads to a positive activity experience and *that* leads to resilient motivation for sustained engagement. Whew! But it's true.

As your Iron Footprint deepens by acquiring content knowledge, your perspective about engagement will mature. This is especially useful when you hit phases where you feel you are not making gains, or when your resilient motivation takes a dip. Phases can be triggered by factors out of our control. For example, ageing's impact on engagement is a reality we all (will likely) encounter. Sore knees, sore shoulders, sore _____ can creep up and mean it's time to retire from running or swimming or _____. This requires an adjustment to engagement, but without the perspective gained from acquiring content knowledge about alternatives, we may think it is the *end* of engagement. Learning how others cope with challenges can help our own transition phases, and this is information that we can gain as content knowledge

Conversely, a lack of content knowledge comparatively diminishes self-confidence, which can lead to regarding engagement as a risky endeavor. Not so much a risk to physical well-being, but to emotional well-being ("I don't think I can do it, therefore I'm not going to try, for I will only fail and disappoint myself"). Engagement from this perspective is approached with psychic hesitancy, second guessing, and uncertainty, and tends to be repetitive from one session to the next. When our routine becomes too routine, we risk the 'justs' -- going through the motions with limited effort. Not only are the results impacted, a downward motivational spiral can be set in motion that can be tough to stem. Ultimately, exercise fatigue weighs heavily because we only consider engaging from a sense of obligation ("I have to do it because it's good for me"). A heavy outlook begets a heavy outlook, which begets quitting activity engagement.

But back to the sunshine.

Multiple modes of media are available to develop content knowledge: books, periodicals, scientific journals, web sites, apps, TV, DVDs. For example, the Golf channel offers terrific instructional material and *Sports Science* on ESPN considers and analyzes sport performance according to scientific principles. While it's 'user beware' for any mode accessed, best-sellers or reputably sponsored sites or shows likely will provide scientifically based, accurate information that is devoid of mis-leading, mythological blather. The litmus test is if something seems outrageous, then it likely is!

For your Iron Footprint, notch the content knowledge you accrue by imprinting it as a FitBUBBLE. This may seem challenging at first because it may not seem clear what to recognize as 'knowledge.' Don't over think the process. If you read an article about how to defend a particular sport's offensive strategy and learn something new this is a FitBUBBLE to notch. Similarly, assign value if you pick up a tip about improving your tennis forehand by watching a DVD or added a new exercise to your deltoid routine by going to a website. Consider cog-nitive engagement achievement as broadly as physical engagement achievement. It certainly bears FitBUBBLE recognition if you made the effort to seek information and learned something new.

Emotional Aspects of Engagement

Emotional indices of engagement include your enjoyment of physical activity or specific activities, your physical activity self-confidence, the sense of satisfaction you yield from participating in an activity or com-pleting a workout, and how motivated you feel to engage in activity. Each of these is a variable that you can track for your Iron Footprint by using a self-made scale or from written narratives, in journal or diary form.

Regular reflection about this aspect of engagement can lead to insight otherwise not gained by imprinting physical or cognitive mea-sures. You may discover emotional patterns about your engagement that were previously unknown. For example, you may learn that you look forward to Mondays at the gym, knowing that it will be crowded and full of distraction, or that you loathe Mondays for having to wait for equipment. Or you may learn that you feel more exhausted, thus a greater sense of accomplishment, upon completing kick-boxing class than you do after using the treadmill, and that your trainer is really controlling and refuses to add motor skill practice to the routine.

You might also mine information about your relationship to physi-cal activity that can prove useful when contemplating changes to your routine or activity environment. For example, for reasons that both support and otherwise impact resilient motivation you may contemplate joining a new gym, hiring a new personal trainer or trying a new group fitness class. The insight you glean from tracking your engagement emotions can help determine if your reasoning stems from recognizing opportunity or is a reaction to discouragement. If it's the latter then the source of discouragement needs to be addressed otherwise motivation will be jeopardized. Regular reflection can lead to the insight needed to find a solution to problem.

For your Iron Footprint, notch affective indices of engagement as FitBUBBLES. To start, choose one or two indices to track (e.g., sense of satisfaction of cardio exercise, confidence rating of different forms of activity), and develop either a numeric scale or written journal to capture its measure. Then, establish a tracking schedule that makes sense for you: daily, weekly, activity to activity, and so on. Once you have tracked for a period of time, you likely will be inspired to add other indices to this aspect of your Iron Footprint tracking.

Summary and a Peek Ahead

Your Iron Footprint icon is yours to create. There is no right or wrong as to what it ought to look like. Just as we have unique relationships to physical activity, we also have unique perspectives from which to express it. The point is to showcase your portfolio—all you have done to foster your health-related fitness (your FitBASE) and all you have done to deepen and broaden your engagement (your FitBUBBLES and FitBESTS). Your Iron Footprint gives features and contours to your physical activity achievement which most important can foster resilient motivation to sustain regular engagement.

Keep in mind that with purchase of this book you also gain membership to www.ironfootprintfitness.com that offers an online platform to create your Iron Footprint and various resources to aid your engagement.

Regardless of whether you create your own image or use the online platform, notching your Iron Footprint across the dimensions of engagement that comprise the physical activity enterprise, as well as for cognitive and affective indices, enables you to recognize your achievement. This fosters resilient exercise motivation, which sustains your activity habit.

What becomes of being too busy to exercise?

As our perspective about engagement and achievement transforms, so too does our schedule. We begin to have so much fun doing achievement-oriented physical activity we clear our leisure-time schedule of everything else!

The next section delivers further insight into *why* creating your Iron Footprint icon can help foster resilient motivation to sustain physical activity engagement. This section also explains *how* the Iron Footprint Fitness approach to considering engagement and recognizing achievement can help to frame activity sessions. Just as the greater your content knowledge about physical activity the more likely your resilient engagement motivation, the more you understand *why and how* the Iron Footprint Fitness approach can enhance and frame your engagement, the more likely it is that you will use it to your benefit.

PART III

MORE ABOUT WHY YOU SHOULD CREATE YOUR IRON FOOTPRINT ICON AND HOW YOU CAN USE IT

Sustaining the motivation to engage regularly in physical activity can be a challenge. Sadly, it can take more psychic effort just to get to the gym than the physical effort exerted once you are there. Certainly, schedules jammed with family and professional commitments contribute to exercise fatigue. At 6:30 p.m., after a stressful day at work and realizing there is no milk at home, getting to the gym becomes second to surviving the grocery store among the others who have realized there is no milk at home. But misguided notions about the realm of physical activity, in particular one's conception of success, might influence exercise fatigue even more.

Reasons notwithstanding, for the sake of our physical well-being, and our very quality of life, we don't have a choice. We need to be physically active—the more the better—and preferably daily.

Iron Footprint Fitness offers a solution to counteract the health-jeopardizing exercise fatigue. Its purpose is to present an approach to physical activity engagement that will transform, invigorate, and refresh your desire to engage, but its primary intent is to foster resilient motivation that will sustain an unwavering commitment to engagement.

Resilient motivation is characterized by hope and autonomy. Iron Footprint Fitness, via the creation of your Iron Footprint icon, depicts your physical activity portfolio, comprised of the multi-dimensions that make up the enterprise of physical activity. An Iron Footprint icon is the mechanism that displays the success that you have achieved in physical activity. A consistent pattern of engagement, adding to your portfolio by trying new activities, and setting performance benchmarks are all examples of achievement. By accessing the success you are realizing, your hope for continued success strengthens. In addition, you internalize your physical self-identity as a proficient performer—"I *am* strong, I *am* a runner, I *can* do motor skills." Optimism and self-identity underlie hope and autonomy, and work in tandem to sustain your motivation to continue regular engagement in physical activity.

Your Iron Footprint icon displays the success you achieve, which you otherwise would miss by looking for what you are not going to find. Radical body transformation, especially how it is fantasized, is unrealistic. Yet it is what can erroneously drive our physical activity engagement, at least until the frustration and despair that result from not realizing the (un-realizable) transformation erode our motivation. By overlooking the good that *is* occurring for results that are likely *never* going to occur, it's no wonder that exercise fatigue and the insidious gremlins overwhelm us like unchecked weeds in a garden. Dejectedly, we stop trying to try.

Creating your Iron Footprint icon breathes sunshine into your relationship with physical activity by transforming your approach to engagement and consideration of how to recognize achievement so that resilient motivation to sustain activity is strengthened. Its building blocks embody attributes of hope and autonomy.

Your Iron Footprint:

CREATES EXCITEMENT about physical activity participation because:

- Success begets success.
  Success is self-generating. Realizing success through notching progress and improvement profoundly nourishes motivation to sustain physical activity engagement and realize further success. By broadly considering achievement as that which occurs across the three dimensions that comprise the physical activity enterprise, multiple opportunities exist to note success.
- Seeing is believing.
  Your success is covertly displayed, and on a frequent basis. This is important because we don't regularly 'see' wellness-marker improvement—e.g., blood pressure, cholesterol, or bone density—so otherwise seeing evidence of achievement makes the esoteric real ("I *am* stronger! I *do* have more endurance! I *am* learning new activities! I *am* achieving!")
- The aspect of *novelty* is added into your routine.
  Being creatures of habit, gym routines can quickly become too routine. Purposefully trying new activities and attempting to set performance benchmarks consistently add variety to weekly, if not daily engagement. Both the novel activity and the anticipation of engaging in the novel activity sustain excitement about engagement. Novel activity also provides something to look forward to.
- Imprinting your icon is cause for celebration.
  Each imprint that is added to your icon represents a physical activity success. Considering how important success is to resilient motivation, imprints are cause for celebration. Celebrating your imprints, or selected imprints, offers an additional layer of recognition. Single layer cake is good, but double layer cake can satisfy more. Acknowledging imprints with a celebratory routine is self-generating. The more you celebrate, the more you want to celebrate, and the more hopeful you are that you will be able to continue to celebrate.
- You can inspire others as well to strive for their personal bests.

Playing your successes forward, meaning inspiring others to track performance benchmarks, is exciting because it simply feels good to know that you have helped someone. But it also stirs your own effort. Likely not openly, but certainly fine if it is, activity engagement naturally arouses comparison. Seeing another person realize a success can instill confidence that you, too, can realize the same. You can share someone's excitement about doing their best time, and then use this energy to go after your own best time.

INCREASES YOUR CONFIDENCE related to physical activity participation and your physical self by:

- Showing evidence of your improvement.
Seeing *that* you are and *how* you are stronger, more flexible, and more skilled, and have greater endurance, is a source of confidence.
- Showing evidence of your growing portfolio.
It's one thing to be interested in trying new activities; it's another to experience new activities. Like attempting anything new, trying new activities can be inherently risky. But the result is satisfaction and a stroke to confidence just for overcoming the risk of trying. This propels you to continue to try new activities. As the (modified) saying goes: "A body stretched by a new experience can never return to its old shape."
- Fostering your identity as an athlete.
Notching success shows evidence that you are a capable and competent activity engager, characteristics that are shared by those who identify as athletes. Declaring as an athlete means that a certain degree of engagement competency has been realized, for taking on an identity requires tangible evidence that we belong. Like someone who makes a successful béarnaise sauce for the first time feeling, "I *am* a chef!" or someone who successfully codes a computer program for the first time feeling, "I *am* a programmer!", the achievement that

46

paved entree into the identity instills confidence that further success is possible. And the identification itself can influence subsequent behavior, for now as a chef I ought to do this or as a programmer I ought to do that. Identifying as an athlete can all the more influence behavior that enhances well-being, for now I ought to consider lifestyle choices. Athletes don't smoke; time for me to quit. Athletes fuel their bodies with nutrient-dense food; time for me to give up junk food. Taking on the identity self-generates the mindset and behavior that characterizes the identity. Me an athlete? *Yes, I am* an athlete, and as an athlete I know that I am capable of realizing further success!

- Uncovering a previously unknown activity-related personal characteristic.

  As the imprinting process unfolds and you experience more and different types of engagement and at a greater level of intensity, you are apt to discover that you possess certain activity-related strengths. Perhaps you realize that you have formidable leg strength, or joint flexibility, or kick-boxing skills. This fuels your self-confidence about activity engagement and strengthens your activity identity.

INSPIRES YOUR EFFORT while engaged in physical activity **by***:*

- Prompting engagement that is intense enough to reap achievement.

  Having tangible benchmarks to reach for leads to more tangible benchmarks to reach for. Our adrenaline is pumped as we attempt to set a personal best, which invokes effort at an intensity not previously realized. Since success begets success, we crave further achievement once success is realized. Tangible benchmarks provide the target, and craving repeated target hits feeds your intensity capacity.

- Engaging with sufficient effort to hit performance benchmarks can also stave off performance plateaus that can occur as your body adapts to the stresses of engagement. Because of the remarkable ability of the human body to respond to the stresses endured during engagement (make gains), different stresses should be introduced periodically, or subsequent gains are unlikely. Consistently striving to hit performance benchmarks inherently means that we engage with optimal effort. We push to hit benchmarks; our body responds; we push further to hit additional benchmarks.

- Reducing or eliminating the 'just' activity sessions.
  Tangible benchmarks are cause for purposeful and intentional activity engagement. This helps to ensure that you engage in activity with sufficient effort or intensity to reap benefit. 'Just' sessions tend to checkmark the "Yes, I did activity today" box, but since the engagement intensity is light, they contribute little to eliciting benefit. Too many 'justs' and any gain made to strengthen your resilient motivation risks being lost to frustration and disappointment.

- Legitimizing the reason for the effort, especially when faced with challenging life circumstances.
  Considering work, family, and other commitments, at some level physical activity engagement might be regarded as gratuitous. Even aware of its fundamental impact on our very quality of life, we may see the gym as discretionary if there is a sick child at home or looming project at work. Then, while there, understandably, any of these gnawing circumstances can dampen the treadmill walk or session of weight training. This is not to suggest that responsibilities be subverted; indeed, the greater our strength (literally and figuratively), the greater our capacity to care for others or manage our workload. The intentionality that this approach offers might be especially useful when your engagement is complicated by 'life.' You can drive the plan, no more/no less, and be assured that it's what you need and ought to do toward your wellness.

- Providing a distraction to the daily routine.
  Even the most highly motivated can experience activity effort that ebbs and flows; it's only natural, and part of being human. Sometimes, routines can become too routine. The same

people, same equipment, same shoes, same play list can be just too same, and even when we make adjustments, lethargy can momentarily set in. Striving to imprint your Iron Footprint Fitness icon across the dimensions of engagement that comprise the enterprise provides a natural distraction from the routine, as the process of imprinting requires that you consistently introduce new facets to your engagement. While you may retain mainstays within your routine, knowing that you are going to be doing something new later is a distraction that can sustain your effort during the whole session.

FOCUSES YOUR PHYSICAL ACTIVITY ENGAGEMENT by:

- Offering purpose to your routine.
  Focusing on specific aspects of achievement offers a way to organize daily workout routines and recreational pursuits. This focus ensures the purpose and meaning of activity sessions, which can stave off an approach from the 'just' perspective, as in, "Today, I'm just going to do some cardio" or "Today, I'm just going to do a few weights." 'Just' sessions tend to be unfocused and meaningless, increasing the likelihood that the outcome yield will be haphazard at best, which jeopardizes motivation.
- Providing accurate assessment that can be used to inform session planning.
  Tracking your performance benchmarks provides an accurate record of assessment. Once you are into the routine of tracking, you may find that certain markers are more stubborn to impact than others. Due to genetics, for example, improving your flexibility may require comparatively more attention, or more than you had anticipated. Without accurate assessment, you may have thought this, but with accurate assessment you can confirm your suspicion. This information can be used to inform how you plan for subsequent activity sessions.

DEVELOPS YOUR PHYSICAL ACTIVITY PERSONALITY by:

- Impressing your Iron Footprint across all dimensions of the physical activity enterprise.
  The more and different ways you experience physical activity, the more deeply your physical activity self is developed, and the more likely it is that your motivation to engage in regular activity is sustained. Impressing your Iron footprint is the means to seeing your physical activity personality blossom. This will empower you to confidently pursue further achievement or experience new activities.
  Having a thin profile jeopardizes your motivation and risks others framing your activity personality. If the offerings of a gym are the only activities you experience, your physical activity personality will be narrowly framed by that gym's programming. If this is the only activity opportunity available, then so be it, but if that isn't the case, avoid the gym defining your physical activity personality. It ought to contribute to your Iron footprint, but not *be* it.

Note – scientists who study aspects of behavior related to physical activity engagement have uncovered principles that when followed increase the likelihood of adhering to regular exercise. Please see *Exercise Adherence and Iron Footprint Fitness* located in Part IV of this book or as a download on www.ironfootprintfitness.com for a description of how the Iron Footprint approach aligns to the principles.

Summary and a Peek Ahead

The attributes of hope and autonomy, critical to developing resilient engagement motivation, are inherent to Iron Footprint Fitness's generous consideration for how achievement ought to be measured and acknowledged. Engaging in activity as Iron Footprint Fitness can also create excitement, inspire your effort and the development of your activity personality and increase your engagement focus and confidence.

The next section offers topic-specific information about the innovative features of Iron Footprint Fitness and helps your transition to the approach. Included are snapshot descriptions of the protocol required to yield health-protection from engagement, and how the approach aligns to principles known to increase the likelihood of adherence to an exercise routine. Also provided are practical suggestions for how to include motor skill practice into your routine, how to begin to organize FitBEST trials, why competition should be embraced, why activity engagement ought to considered from an 'every day' perspective, and what is realistic to expect regarding body transformation that can result from engagement.

The topics apply to anyone adopting Iron Footprint Fitness and help shift engagement accordingly. Additional topics are available as White Paper downloads at the Iron Footprint Fitness Academy of Ironfootprintfitness.com. Among others, these include *Seniors and Iron Footprint Fitness*, *KidPRINT*, and *Technology and Iron Footprint Fitness.*

PART IV

THE INNOVATIVE FEATURES OF IRON FOOTPRINT FITNESS AND SPECIAL TOPICS RELATED TO ADOPTING THE APPROACH

This section presents several essays that distinguish the uniqueness of the Iron Footprint Fitness approach to engagement within the fitness/health genre. Toward offering a solution to inconsistent motivation to engage in activity, Iron Footprint Fitness:

- Introduces the concept of *engagement-resilient motivation*
- Introduces the concept of *achievement-oriented health-related fitness*
- Presents physical activity as a *multi-dimensional enterprise* consisting of different types of engagement
- Introduces Iron Footprint as a platform to showcase activity achievement according to the engagement dimensions of *FitBASE, FitBESTS, and FitBUBBLES*

- Introduces *motor-skill practice* as a regular component of FitBASE (daily) engagement

In addition, Iron Footprint Fitness is:

- Free of cost – doesn't require the purchase of equipment, DVD's, special clothes, etc.
- Agile – adaptable (and effective) to anyone regardless of age, gender, exercise history, degree of skill proficiency, gym members, home-exercisers, and whether using a personal trainer or not

The narratives will help you better understand the innovative features. The topics include why approaching physical activity as Iron Footprint Fitness can lead to resilient motivation, how you need to engage in activity to yield health protection, how to organize your engagement for motor skill practice and FitBEST trials, why competition can be a good thing, what is realistic body transformation to expect from engagement, and the importance of considering activity from a simple perspective.

To begin, a picture of Iron Footprint Fitness's *Power of "ER"* for how the flavor of this type of engagement is different from non-Iron Footprint Fitness engagement and why this is important to your activity motivation.

The Power of "ER": StrongER Than Before…FastER Than Before…FarthER Than Before…BettER Than Before…OftenER Than Before

Regular physical activity is the foundation for developing optimal physical (and emotional) wellness and contributing to our quality of life. No secret—we know this—and on the days when our motivation cooperates, we juice up our iPods for a walk or go to the gym to lift a few weights or take a group fitness class.

Good. But could it be better?

There is a big difference between daily physical activity and DAILY PHYSICAL ACTIVITY—it's the factor of "ER"—for both its pursuit and its capture.

Daily physical activity can be kind of milquetoast, beige, average, conciliatory, "C" work, passing. There's nothing really wrong with what we are doing; it meets minimum requirements. It's acceptable.

But DAILY PHYSICAL ACTIVITY that pursues "ER" can be exhilarating, impassioned, and fun, and most important, capturing an "ER" fosters engagement motivation. An "ER" is an engagement achievement. It marks the occasion when some aspect of our engagement has been strongER, fastER, farthER, or bettER than ever, significant because success motivates subsequent engagement by offering hope that further success is possible. In hope there is optimism, perseverance, and energy. With hope, we are excited about today's engagement and already looking forward to tomorrow's.

Iron Footprint Fitness approaches engagement from the "ER" perspective, and FitBASE, FitBUBBLES, and FitBESTS display its capture. This approach promotes DAILY PHYSICAL ACTIVITY that fosters a level of physical robustness unlikely through daily physical activity, and the hope that more is possible. The resilient motivation that is developed sustains regular activity, which cultivates wellness. For this, the merit of an "ER" approach speaks loudly. After all, our quality of life stands to be more than beige, average, "C" work, or just passing, and it's with "ER" that we can transform our degree of motivation to GRRR!

. . .

Iron Footprint Fitness and Strategies to Increase Exercise Adherence

The first week of January brings the hope of a new year. It also brings crowds to the gym not seen since the previous first week in January. The newly exercise resolute—those who have resolved to get more exercise—excitedly figure out how to use the treadmill and manipulate free weights. The regulars take waiting for equipment in stride, knowing it's only a matter of time before the novelty wears off and most stop coming. By the end of January, the gym's landscape will be back to normal, until the cycle repeats itself the following January.

Why do some stick to their exercise routine, while others do not?

Exercise adherence research has uncovered strategies that increase the likelihood of sustainment to an exercise routine. For the purpose specific to Iron Footprint Fitness, adherence is considered broadly to include all forms of physical activity engagement, not just formal exercise.

The following strategies increase the likelihood of adhering to engagement. Since their complexity bears description that ranges beyond this narrative, the premise of each focuses upon its alignment to Iron Footprint Fitness.

Engage in Exercises (Activity) You Enjoy

The realm of physical activity is comprised of multiple forms of movement, each capable of yielding health protection and allowing the unique expression of your physical self. The form of movement you engage in should be enjoyable!

The more clustered your FitBUBBLES, the greater your repertoire of engagement, and the more likely you have experienced and assessed multiple forms of movement for appeal. Through the process of impressing FitBUBBLES, engagement likes and dislikes are fine-tuned. This is valuable self-discovery even if the results are not necessarily surprising:"I tried Zumba, but I don't care for dance, so I didn't like it." It deepens your understanding of your physical self, which clarifies your engagement autonomy and provides engagement peace of mind. The more FitBUBBLES you cluster, the more you assure enjoyable engagement choices.

Utilize a Choice of Activities

Your FitBASE routine can be self-generating—the more you do the routine, the more the routine becomes a habit. The habit of engagement is key to well-being, but you need to avoid your routine becoming monotonous, or too routine. Engaging in a variety of activities can stave off boredom, stagnation, and effort from a "just" approach ("Today I'm going to *just* do a little cardio" or "Today I'm going to *just* lift a few weights."). It can also decrease the risk of developing over-use injuries.

Choice itself is empowering. Choosing your engagement activity creates a much stronger connection to the activity than being told what to do or going through the motions of what you always do. Choice conjures anticipation, which (hopefully) guarantees that enjoyment will result. An excited "I get to __ today at the gym" approach is more conducive to sustainability than a glum "I have to __ today at the gym" approach, even knowing how important what you "have to do" is for your well-being.

The more clustered your FitBUBBLES, the more successful this strategy. Possessing the capacity to engage in many different forms of activity means more options. Clustering FitBUBBLES strengthens the relationship you have with your physical self and results in a repertoire of activities from which you can choose to engage on any given day. This increases the likelihood of sustained engagement motivation.

Base Goals on Time, Not Distance, and Set Them Yourself

Self-generated goals increase the likelihood of a strong connection to the purpose of engagement. If left to the influence of others, e.g., personal trainers, purpose can seem otherworldly, which can erode effort. Feeling "made to" do something can trigger rebellion against it.

One challenge to goal setting is the lack of information about current performance measures. This is remedied by impressing FitBESTS—performance benchmarks and markers of physical wellness. This is accurate information you can be use to set relevant performance goals (e.g., increase upper body strength, increase hamstring flexibility) and wellness goals (e.g., lower blood pressure, develop leaner body composition). FitBEST impression also generates a constant flow of information that can be used to adjust goals when necessary.

Tracking distance can be a deceiving goal. Completing a certain distance during engagement (i.e. three miles of running or walking) does not guarantee health-related impact, which instead requires exercising at your target heart rate for a certain amount of time. If the distance completed is for the appropriate amount of time at your target heart rate, then health-related benefit is likely, but this leaves much to chance. Focusing solely upon covering a distance during engagement risks diminished achievement compared to exercising for a set amount of time. This can stress motivation, if not erode it over time.

Approaching engagement from the Iron Footprint perspective tracks achievement in terms of both time and distance variables, as well as when it represents having done extra activity on a given day. For example, FitBEST markers can easily be established to acknowledge the longest distance ever walked/run/cycled and time trials for specified distances (e.g., one mile, 5K, 10K, marathon, half-century, century), and FitBUBBLES can also be impressed if the distance covered was separate or in addition to FitBASE engagement.

Focus on the Environment Rather than Your Body during Exercise to Reduce Boredom and Fatigue

Distract yourself from the process of FitBASE engagement with music, TV, DVDs, and conversation with your exercise neighbor to divert your attention away from routines that can become monotonous. Simply knowing that distractions are available can ease the stress that arises from anticipating the dullness that arises from repetition.

Iron Footprint Fitness engagement reduces the likelihood of boredom by expecting that FitBASE routines will be augmented with novel activities (e.g., motor skill practice, attempting a FitBEST trial, doing a new activity to add a FitBUBBLE.). Novel activities generate excitement at doing something unique or different from the everyday. Attempting a FitBEST or adding a FitBUBBLE stirs adrenaline, which combats the sameness of the routine. Engagement freshness is sustained by adhering to a regular schedule of attempting benchmarks or trying new activities, and adding motor skill practice to your routine.

Keep Exercise Logs

Exercise logs display a record of participation. Tangible evidence of engagement nourishes the desire to keep adding to the record.

An Iron Footprint both logs engagement *and* displays engagement achievement for how it occurs across the dimensions of the physical activity enterprise: daily routine (FitBASE), performance benchmarks (FitBESTS), and accumulation of physical activity (FitBUBBLES).

Choose Purposeful and Meaningful Activities

Physical activity encompasses a multitude of movement forms. Some are especially useful for promoting health-related fitness, while others are valued for triggering personal meaning. Motivation is enhanced when the chosen activity matches the purpose of engagement, and when it is movement that carries personal meaning.

Health protection requires engagement geared toward cardiovascular and muscular strength, and endurance and joint flexibility. Activities need to yield these outcomes effectively, and engagement needs to be appropriately intense to stimulate gains. Your Iron Footprint displays performance capacity that can be used to ensure that engagement is appropriately intense to yield health-related benefit (i.e. using adequate resistance during weight training). Tracking your engagement also provides a record of progress to determine when to make adjustments to activity choices or intensity levels.

Intentionally seeking to impress your Iron Footprint also frames the purpose of engagement for any given session, be it health protection (FitBASE), performance benchmarks (FitBEST), or deepening your activity profile by trying a new activity or engaging in an activity other than your routine (FitBUBBLE).

Impressing Iron Footprint FitBUBBLES deepens your physical-activity portfolio, which enables you to discern your engagement likes and dislikes. The more forms of movement you have tried, the more you will discover what is especially meaningful to you and the reason for the connection. For example, you may find that you like softball because you like to hit things, or that you have come to like surfing because you like the way it feels to glide on water. You also may discover that you like an activity for the simple reason that you are good at it or have been able to become proficient quickly. This insight can be mined because the knowledge that you engaged in more activity than your FitBASE routine is as valuable as impressing the FitBUBBLES. Gleaning the reason why an activity appeals to you feeds your desire to keep engaging in the activity. This loops to impressing more FitBUBBLES, which means accruing more activity. Net/net, the likelihood for enhanced well-being improves.

Reward Yourself for Attendance, Participation, and Goals Met

Rewards can help sustain adherence by providing tangible incentives to recognize attendance and performance achievement. Having a reward to shoot for provides an end to the means of engagement different from enjoyment or health protection. We sustain engagement because it is fun and fosters our well-being, but we can also earn a prize! This nourishes the part of our psyche that lights up at the chance to earn something. A reward system can both entice engagement and be its means of celebration.

Through notching FitBASE, FitBESTS, and FitBUBBLES, Iron Footprint offers an intuitive method to capture attendance and participation *and* important details *about* participation.

Attendance merits recognition, as engagement benefit is obviously otherwise impossible. Regular engagement is an achievement to be acknowledged, but Iron Footprint Fitness suggests that it is beneficial to establish a realistic reward mark toward the realization of health-related fitness gain. Although each FitBASE routine can enhance our well-being, measured improvement requires sustained engagement (e.g., improving one-repetition maximum bench press, improving blood pressure, improving hamstring flexibility). A minimum of 16 FitBASE sessions a month (four per week) is reasonable toward inducing improvement. Your attendance reward follows after notching your 16th FitBASE session of each month.

FitBUBBLES can be used to structure rewards for other aspects of engagement. The prize structure could reward each notched FitBUBBLE equally or be scaled to reward especially meaningful FitBUBBLES more (e.g, taking swimming lessons though fearful of water, summoning the nerve to join pickup basketball at the park, volunteering at a school's physical education class).

FitBESTS can structure how to reward participation for performance quality. This can include goals that are met or benchmarks that are set, each being an intuitive indicator of achievement and appropriate to reward. Similar to FitBUBBLE recognition, the prize structure for FitBESTS could reward each equally or be scaled to reward tiered achievement. Iron Footprint recommends rewarding each FitBEST for the initial roll-out of this incentive strategy.

Reward Ideas

The reward scheme or prize structure you establish depends upon your interests within and outside of physical activity and your budget. The incentive is only as strong as your value of the reward. To be most effective, rewards ought to be something special, outside the realm of your everyday experience. Reward ideas are as follows:

Physical activity-themed rewards (enjoy the reward you have earned *and* add a FitBUBBLE): tickets to a professional sporting event, new gym shoes or workout apparel, extra sessions with a sport-teaching professional (e.g, golf or tennis lessons), massage, day pass to a different gym, downloads for your iPod mixed to match your engagement tempo, a session of activity/equipment rental (e.g., kayaking, paddleboarding, skiing, roller-skating/blading, ice skating, rock climbing, bowling), a piece of sports equipment (e.g., new glove, new tennis racquet).

Non-physical activity focused rewards: movie, theater, concert, performance, dinner out.

Reward ideas for a limited budget: family member doing your house chores or cooking you dinner, new socks, new shoelaces, new lifting gloves, special dinner at home (e.g., fresh lobster or cut of meat).

Reward yourself accordingly, but not with a day off. Cheers to the celebration!

Focus on the Present, the Process, and the Experience— Exercise for Its Own Sake, Not Just toward Some Future Gain

Physical activity enhances life quality for reasons other than well-being. For example, engagement is inherently a good way to spend time; it is also fun, a means of social camaraderie, and a manner of self-expression. The process of engagement can be as worthwhile as the yielded product. Enjoying the piped music at the gym the company of fellow exercisers, or the antics of teammates has value for what each contributes to the engagement experience.

FitBUBBLES can be impressed for aspects of engagement different from performance achievement or health protection. Recognizing cognitive (mental) and affective (emotional) factors can help you gain perspective and capture the essence of the whole of engagement. For example, taking the time to research the correct way to dribble a basketball enhances your content knowledge, which can lead to even more purposeful engagement. The content knowledge you gain ought to be acknowledged as a FitBUBBLE, as it grows your activity portfolio. Creating the means to chronicle process aspects of your engagement experience also contributes to your activity portfolio. Written journals or reflections that focus upon the experience itself (e.g., a scaled assessment of what was fun, a narrative that describes the antics of teammates) are artifacts that capture yet more aspects of engagement. Whether you decide to recognize these as FitBUBBLES (see Part II to review how to recognize affective aspects of engagement as FitBUBBLES) or leave them as stand-alone entries, their capture impresses your Iron Footprint, for it enhances your understanding of engagement.

The Fitter You Are, the More Likely You Will Sustain Regular Exercise

Success begets success, which leads to further success.

Seeking to impress your Iron Footprint encourages you to improve your engagement capacity (FitBASE and FitBESTS), which leads to improved measures of health-related fitness. This achievement leads to hope that more is possible, which helps to sustain regular engagement.

Self-efficacy Is Critical to Transform from Being Sedentary to Sustaining Regular Engagement

Self-efficacy (self-confidence) is the belief we have in our ability to engage in activity successfully. The strongest source of engagement self-efficacy is past performance. If we have experienced success in the past, we believe that we can continue to be successful and will be excited to engage again. But if we have not been successful, we tend not to be motivated to engage again.

Seeking to impress your Iron Footprint encourages you to improve your engagement capacity. This means, for example, getting stronger, developing greater endurance and learning, or honing motor skills. Capturing your achievement displays evidence that you *have* been successful, which motivates you to continue to engage. This ultimately helps the transformation from someone who is habitually sedentary to someone who sustains regular engagement.

Summary

Engagement motivation is a complex concept, but certain principles have been uncovered through research that increase the likelihood of sticking to a regular habit. Approaching engagement from the Iron Footprint Fitness perspective complements the principles for how the approach encourages multidimensional achievement and for how subsequent achievement is documented for display.

Note: The compilation of strategies is sourced from the reference listed below. Please access this book to learn more about the psychology of sport and exercise engagement. Knowledge is power, and this book provides a wealth of information that can be uniquely useful toward helping you sustain engagement and impress your Iron Footprint. Also keep in mind that the content knowledge you acquire can be acknowledged as a FitBUBBLE.

Reference

Weinberg, R. and D. Gould. *Foundations of Sport and Exercise Psychology.* 5th ed. Human
    Kinetics: Champaign, IL, 2011.

· · ·

Achievement-Oriented Health-Related Fitness: What We Need to Know

*"Physical activity can be health protective when
achievement-oriented, health-related engagement is the daily habit."*
-Iron Footprint Fitness

Ancient civilizations considered regular, vigorous physical activity essential toward developing optimal quality of life. Fast-forward several millennia, and the sentiment is now scientific—*physical activity can be health protective!* This notion is not lost on the vast majority of us, nor is the notion that playing sports or otherwise engaging in exercise is fun and an inherently good way to spend time. However, less than half of American adults engage in enough physical activity to elicit health benefits (United States Department of Health and Human Services), which has contributed to obesity and obesity-related health care costs in the billions and projected to triple over the next decades (Centers for Disease Control and Prevention). While we may agree with the notion of activity's benefit, it seems less clear *why* it is good, what the specific benefits are, and what is required for the benefits to be realized. What follows outlines the health-related benefit that physical activity can yield *and* describes what's required of engagement to ensure that it is health protective.

To begin, physical well-being is a product of our cardiovascular and muscular proficiency, joint range of motion, and body composition (ratio of body fat tissue to lean [muscle] tissue). Taken together, the health-related benefit that physical activity can yield falls within the categories of *cardiovascular health*, *muscular strength and muscular endurance*, *flexibility*, and *body composition*. These are also known as the components of health-related fitness.

More specifically, regular physical activity can yield the following measures of health protection:

- Healthy blood pressure
- Healthy blood sugar (reduced risk of diabetes)
- Healthy body weight (reduced risk of overweight)
- Healthy percentage of body fat (reduced risk of obesity)
- Healthy bone density (reduced risk of osteoporosis)
- Reduced risk of certain cancers
- Healthy cholesterol (reduced risk of heart attack, stroke)
- Healthy blood flow
- Enhanced self-esteem from maintaining a routine and realizing performance improvement
- The release of endorphins that elicit the "runner's high"
- Cognitive integrity
- Enhanced mood stability from releasing stress
- Eased anxiety and depression

Next, a few points of clarity before moving forward:

First, "health-related" fitness is different from "performance-related" fitness. Health-related fitness is engagement that yields health protection. Performance-related fitness includes attributes of movement that complement athletic proficiency: agility, power, quickness, foot speed, and so on. Being able to throw a ball proficiently, an attribute of performance, in and of itself will not yield health protection.

Second, health-protective engagement is not exclusive to the athletically gifted. Health-related fitness and athletic proficiency can be, but are *not* necessarily, synonymous. Realizing the health benefit of engagement is possible regardless of the ability to throw, catch, or kick a ball. Skill proficiency can help sustain a regular engagement habit (which is one reason Iron Footprint Fitness introduces skill practice as a FitBASE component), but it's not required to obtain health protection.

Third, a formal background in kinesiology or exercise science is not required to understand the underlying concepts of health-related fitness or to understand what engagement requirements yield health-related benefit.

Last, not all physical activity is the same. Engagement that yields health protection is different than leisure engagement, because health protection is dependent upon engaging according to the principles that yield achievement. While some engagement is always better than no engagement, leisure activities tend to be of low intensity (e.g., a casual stroll in the park), not vigorous enough to yield optimum benefit.

To illustrate, the Centers for Disease Control (CDC) outlines the engagement parameters that are adequate to yield health protection. While daily engagement is best, the *minimum* guidelines are these:

- 150 minutes of moderate aerobics (cardiovascular exercise) per week and two strength training* days per week, or
- 75 minutes of vigorous aerobics and two strength training* days per week, or
- a mix of moderate and vigorous aerobics and two strength training* days per week.

  *Minimum strength training is completing one set of eight to 12 repetitions for each major muscle group.

To yield *greater* benefit, the guidelines are as follows:

- 300 minutes of moderate aerobics per week and two strength training days per week, or
- 150 minutes of vigorous aerobics per week and two strength training days per week.

Iron Footprint Fitness advocates a consistent pattern of FitBASE engagement, but one that is also sufficiently intense to yield health benefit. *Achievement-oriented health-related fitness* is introduced herein to describe the protocol that is required to gain benefit in each health-related fitness component. The intent is to convey key information about *achieving* within each component to ensure that your FitBASE routine *is* health-protective.

Cardiovascular Strength

Anchored by the heart muscle, the cardiovascular system pumps blood and controls respiration. The healthier the heart, the more efficiently blood is pumped, with optimal volume and pressure. Like other muscles, the heart requires exertion to sustain its strength. Engaging in "aerobic" physical activity yields heart health, but the exertion needs to be appropriately intense. Too much increases the risk for injury, while not enough fails to stimulate benefit. Intensity is measured by heart rate during engagement, and a simple formula determines your appropriate heart-rate training zone:

220 minus your age (maximum heart rate), then take 65 to 75 percent (heart-rate training zone) of that number.

For example, a 50-year-old's maximum heart rate is 170 beats per minute (220 − 50), but his or her heart-rate training zone is between 110 (65% of maximum) and 127 (75% of maximum) beats per minute. The low end of the training zone is considered moderate intensity, and the high end of the training zone is considered vigorous intensity.

Many different types of activity can be "aerobic": walking, running, cycling, spinning, group aerobics (e.g., step, kickboxing, jazzercise), elliptical, StairMaster or stair mill, swimming, rowing, circuit training, skating (in-line or ice), and skiing (especially cross-country). The movement form doesn't matter so long as a safely elevated heart rate is sustained for the recommended duration of time to foster cardiovascular benefit—a minimum of 150 minutes of moderate, or 75 minutes of vigorous, aerobic physical activity a week, or for greater cardiovascular benefit, 300 minutes of moderate or 150 minutes of vigorous activity a week. Considering the benefit, *daily* cardiovascular activity ought to be prioritized.

Note: Aerobic activity can be done in chunks, but it has to be at a vigorous intensity for at least 10 minutes to reap benefit.

How to measure your heart rate during exercise:
1. Purchase and use a heart-rate monitor. Available at most well-stocked sporting goods stores, some models offer basic functions, while others include sophisticated features. Choose the model you are comfortable with, and read the directions

thoroughly so you will understand the meaning of the readout number(s). Gaze at the readout during your engagement, and adjust your intensity (effort) as necessary to stay within your heart-rate training zone.

2. Use the time readout on the piece of cardio equipment you are using. There are two ways to monitor your heart rate using this method:

   Note: Use your index and middle fingers in tandem to determine your heart rate. Do not use your thumb.

   a. Count your heart rate for 10 seconds, then multiply that number by six to determine your beats per minute. First, find your pulse, either along your neck (carotid artery) or directly on your heart. (I find the heart location to have the stronger pulse.) Begin your count with one when the time readout shows any number ending with one (one, 11, 21, 31, 41, 51), then end your count when the readout reaches the subsequent number ending with zero (e.g., if you begin your count at one, end your count at 10; if you begin your count at 11, end your count at 20; if you begin your count at 21, end your count at 30). Multiply that number by six to determine your heart rate for one minute.

   b. Count your heart rate for six seconds, then add a zero to that number to determine your beats per minute. Begin your count when the time readout shows any number ending with one (see above), then end your count when the readout reaches the subsequent number ending with six (e.g, if you begin your count at one, end your count at six; if you begin your count at 11, end your count at 16; if you begin your count at 21, end your count at 26). Then, add a zero to the number to determine your heart rate for one minute.

Note: Most pieces of cardio equipment come equipped with a heart-rate feature. Users hold sensors for a certain period of time until heart rate is displayed. While the readout *may* be accurate, either of the methods described above can ensure accuracy. Appropriate exertion is critical toward reaping cardio-vascular benefit. Don't rely on what *might* be accurate.

Points of Physical Reality

In name of cardio, exercisers often engage until covering a certain distance or a completing a certain amount of time, but this does not ensure optimal cardiovascular gain unless it is accomplished for a sufficient duration at the appropriate intensity. Otherwise, walking on the treadmill means just that, walking on the treadmill.

Aiming to cover a certain distance or to cover a distance in a certain time, as well as 'extra' activity outside of your FitBASE routine, can imprint your Iron Footprint as a FitBEST or FitBUBBLE, but simply walking on the treadmill for a prescribed distance or time period won't yield optimum benefit unless you do it with appropriate intensity.

Exercise your heart, but do so to *achieve* optimum benefit. All physical activity is not the same. Carefully adhere to these guiding principles to foster your heart health.

Muscular Strength and Muscular Endurance

In concert with the central nervous system, skeletal muscles pull against bones to produce movement. Muscles also enable posture and protect vital organs, and muscular capacity can profoundly impact quality of life for its contribution to robustness, vitality, and independence. The more muscular strength and endurance we possess, the easier it is to go about the physical tasks common to daily life: getting in and out of the car, getting up and out of chairs, shuttling kids to school, grocery shopping, doing the wash, cleaning the house, and so on. Albeit less than for previous generations given advances in mechanism and technology, we all require some degree of muscular strength/endurance to accomplish tasks—the more the better.

Muscular capacity also impacts engagement outside the gym, as well as body composition. The quality with which we hit a softball, return a serve, or throw a football is correlated to strength and endurance, and the greater our ratio of lean mass (muscle tissue) to adipose tissue (fat), the healthier our body composition. Body composition as a health-related fitness component is presented in a forthcoming section, but the muscular capacity that can be developed through weight training is significant for its contribution to metabolism, which impacts your ratio of lean to fat tissue. Both bigger muscles and stronger muscles boost metabolism, which aids in maintaining a healthy body composition.

Improving muscular capacity requires exercises with weights that *overload* muscles by requiring more work than usual to complete a move. Weight training is executed by completing a certain number of repetitions of an exercise for a certain number of times (sets) for each targeted muscle. The key principle is using weight that is heavy enough to overload the muscle. For muscular strength gains, five to seven repetitions of an exercise should be completed, and for muscular endurance gains, 10 to 12 repetitions should be completed. The weight used needs to be *heavy* enough that each set's last repetition is difficult to complete. This is achievement-oriented overload that will stimulate muscular gains. And because muscles are remarkable for their ability to adapt to stresses, progressive stress—heavier and heavier resistance—is needed to stimulate ongoing gains in strength and endurance.

The CDC recommends a minimum of two strength-training days a week, with each major muscle group being targeted for one set of eight to 12 repetitions. The major muscles to target include pectorals (chest), deltoids (shoulders), latissimus dorsi (back), biceps/triceps (arms), quadriceps (front of thigh), gluteus group (buttocks), and hamstrings (back of thigh). At least 48 hours should separate strength-training sessions of any muscle to allow sufficient time for the muscle to regenerate. For example, if pectorals are targeted on Monday, they shouldn't be targeted again until at least Wednesday. Additional muscular benefit can be realized by increasing the number of strength-training sessions per week, or the number of sets completed for each muscle. Considering how important muscular capacity is for quality of life and wellness, Iron Footprint Fitness suggests establishing a weight-training routine that exceeds the minimum recommendation. A fitness professional can help design an achievement-oriented routine that also accounts for the appropriate amount of recovery between working muscle groups.

Points of Physical Reality

Note to women: Due to hormonal differences (comparably less testosterone), women are not capable of gaining the same degree of muscle mass as men (unless chemically augmented). However, achievement-oriented weight training will result in bigger muscles—and this is a *good thing!*

Muscular mass is extremely important for how it contributes to bone density, protects the skeleton, and leads to robustness. Bones are organic matter that require stimulation for density to be generated. The greater the density, the less likely breaks will occur. Bone density is stimulated by muscles pulling against bones, especially as occurring during physical activity. Weight-bearing exercise (e.g., walking, running, forms of group fitness classes) and weight training require muscles to pull against bones for movement to be executed. The more *mass* that pulls against the bone, the more the bone will be stimulated to develop girth.

Weight training to foster strength, endurance, *and* mass can also counteract the impact aging has on bone density. According to the National Osteoporosis Foundation, 25 million Americans are afflicted with osteoporosis, including half of all women over the age of 50. The research is indisputable: achievement-oriented weight training that yields muscular mass can stimulate bone health. As much mass as possible ought to be developed to maintain as much bone density as possible.

Further, most of us would rather look strong than not, but more important than what we look like is how *what we do* to achieve the look contributes to wellness! Robust physiques are developed by achievement-oriented engagement that yields heart health and musculature, and minimizes body fat. Being robust is a good thing, and muscle mass contributes to robustness.

Last, achievement-oriented, health-related weight training does not include outcomes of "shaping," "toning," and/or "contouring." Each implies a goal that grossly neglects the health- impacting development of strength, endurance, and mass. Each also represents the pursuit of ambiguous outcomes—likely never realized—that dangerously jeopardize motivation. While women's response to weight training won't yield the same degree of strength or mass as men due to hormonal makeup, the purpose for doing so is gender neutral.

Flexibility

Movement is greatly influenced by the range of motion of joints and the suppleness of soft tissue (including muscles). Flexibility is the degree to which joints and soft tissue maintain optimal range of motion. Joints that have limited range of motion and muscles that have reduced elasticity compromise the quality of movement.

Efficient physical movement is rhythmic and flowing. Compromised range of motion, "inflexibility," or "tightness" can contribute to movement that is jerky, lopsided, unbalanced, and painful. Range of motion can be limited by neglecting to engage in flexibility exercises, degenerative disease such as arthritis, or damage such as cartilage tears. If you are afflicted by disease or damage, flexibility exercises may not restore your range of motion but can aid in its optimum maintenance.

Flexibility is addressed by engaging in dynamic (moving) and static (not moving) stretching. Dynamic stretching includes movement such as leg pendulum swings (to the front and side), high-knee walking/marching, glute kicks, and big arm circles. Dynamic stretching does not hold poses for a certain amount of time, and is recommended as a warm-up to more intense engagement to promote blood flow and prevent injury. Any bout of moderately vigorous activity should be preceded by two to three minutes of light aerobic activity (e.g., light jog, moderate walk on the treadmill) that is then followed with dynamic stretching.

Static stretching induces the lengthening of muscles by holding poses. A static stretching routine should be done to conclude a physical activity session. Working from the top of the body to the bottom, at minimum, static stretches should be done for the shoulders/chest, arms, front and back of legs, buttocks, and calves. Stretches for each muscle/muscle group should be held for 10 to 20 seconds.

Points of Physical Reality

Mind-body, aesthetic exercising (e.g., yoga, Pilates) has become popular in recent years. While this form of movement yields health-related gains, *only* doing these types will compromise overall health-related achievement. In particular, this type of activity will not yield the same cardiovascular benefit as aerobic activity. At the other end of the spectrum, stretching needs to be a consistent component of your FitBASE routine. At stake is preserving structural alignment and the suppleness of soft tissue, which naturally diminishes through aging. Range of motion will erode more so and be compromised much earlier in life without consistently addressing this health-related fitness component.

Further, the risk of injury increases without regular stretching, which can result in having to take time off from activity. The physical health ramifications are obvious, but perhaps under-considered is the emotional toll that time away can induce. Engagement provides a unique, healthful response to life's stressors—an outcome not to be taken for granted or undervalued. In addition, there is the potential for one-time injuries or annoying conditions to turn into nagging or chronic issues that require professional care if a consistent stretching routine is not followed. For example, 70 to 80 percent of adults experience low-back pain at some point in their lives. Stretching that targets the abdominals and back muscles is commonly considered to both treat and prevent the condition. The pervasiveness alone establishes the need to include stretching as part of your FitBASE routine.

Body Composition

Our bodies are made up of lean tissue (muscle, bones, organs) and adipose tissue (fat). Because of the health-impacting difference between the characteristics of lean and adipose tissue, the greater the ratio of lean mass to fat mass, the (generally) healthier we are.

Achieving healthy body composition requires adherence to the following:

- Balancing food intake with energy expenditure to control body fat and
- Building lean mass

Aerobic exercise and weight training are critical to body composition. Aerobic exercise burns calories and controls body fat. If energy balance is not regulated (calories in equaling calories burned), body weight and body fat increase, and so does the risk for obesity-related disease. Weight training builds lean mass. Growing muscles, *achieving* within the health-related fitness component of muscular capacity, contributes to both muscular-related health and healthy body composition.

Body composition can be measured by fitness professionals using sophisticated equipment. If this is unrealistic, determining your BMI (body mass index, a ratio of body weight relative to height) is a convenient, noninvasive, and reliable alternative. BMI calculators can be accessed on a number of web sites by entering "BMI" into a search engine.

Note: Research has determined that BMI criteria may not be accurate for Asian populations. Additional tests can be conducted to best assess the body composition of members of this population. Seek assistance from a health professional to undergo body composition testing.

Points of Physical Reality

First, accurately determining healthfulness based upon body weight or physical appearance alone is not possible without further assessment to determine body composition. Even if body weight is in the so-called healthy zone (some insurance companies use weight relative to height charts to determine this aspect of health), the composition of the weight may be unhealthy. The opposite can also apply, since muscle weighs more than fat. Those who are heavily muscled tend to weigh more than the healthy zone for their height, which inaccurately renders them unhealthy.

In a related vein, physical appearance can also be deceiving in determining healthfulness. For example, consider two women of the same height who appear to have similar physiques (i.e. wear the same size clothes). One woman, though, weighs 120 pounds and carries 20 percent body fat, while the other weighs 130 pounds and carries 12 percent body fat. All things equal, the heavier woman is generally healthier because her body composition has a greater percentage of lean tissue than the other. (*Note* – a variety of factors contribute to health. The example is meant to illustrate how appearance itself can be a deceiving indicator.)

A second point is using creative license to illustrate the health-impacting, qualitative differences between lean and adipose tissue.

Excess fat is the bullying weed in the garden—it has no redeemable social graces or sense of boundaries, wants attention, and annoyingly seeks it by springing up wherever it can. While its gnarled root system will not ever entirely disappear, it can be hidden underground through consistent effort (regular, health-related physical activity) so as not to subject others to its ugliness. Muscle is the warm sun. It nourishes, stimulates growth, and promotes well-being for what it has the capacity to do—produce movement. Muscle is a giver. Unlike fat cells that are comparatively dormant, muscle cells are active and organic. Muscle cells participate in life because they, themselves, live. Fat cells are Web surfing, video playing, sedentary couch potatoes. Muscles get up and get going, but fat only observes life as it occurs around it.

Summary

We owe it to ourselves to ensure that our FitBASE engagement is *health related* and *achievement oriented*, a routine of exercise that strengthens the heart, strengthens and builds muscles, improves joint range of motion, and improves or sustains healthy body composition.

Abide by the aforementioned *achievement* protocol to yield these health-protective outcomes. Otherwise, underactivity, ineffective activity, and activity that neglects the requirements for health achievement can cost your pocketbook and, most important, your quality of life.

References

1. Centers for Disease Control and Prevention, www.cdc.gov
2. National Osteoporosis Foundation,www.nof.org
3. National Institute of Neurological Disorders and Stroke of the National Institutes of Health, www.ninds.nih.gov
4. United States Department of Health and Human Services, www.hhs.gov

• • •

Add Motor Skill Practice to Your Routine—Why and How?

Motor skill practice? Like dribbling a basketball around cones? Or kicking a soccer ball? Or throwing a football? Or skipping around an obstacle course?

Yes!

The Iron Footprint Fitness notion of "motor skill practice" is the intentional inclusion of locomotor (e.g., skipping, galloping, hopping), non-locomotor (e.g., bending, twisting), and manipulative (e.g., throwing, catching, kicking, dribbling) skill practice during engagement.

In our quest to develop our physical selves, we ought to acquire the ability to move in all manners possible, and to how that movement applies to activity in a variety of different contexts. The relationship we have with our physical selves depends on our movement expression. The more skill we possess and the greater its proficiency, the more activity forms we can engage in, and the deeper our Iron Footprint. Motor skill practice like skipping in a zigzag pattern, galloping in low and high positions, and kicking to targets has merit for the joy it can elicit and its contribution to our Iron Footprint.

Motor-skill acquisition typically is associated with childhood and adolescence, but proficiency can improve throughout the lifespan. Aging can diminish qualities of performance like speed and quickness, but although we lose what we don't use, what we continue to use (or learn to use) will enable us to reduce the loss. It's never too late to learn or refine motor skills even if the performance quality is lesser than during formative years. Much good can emerge from adding this to your routine, including priceless smiles and laughter during its practice.

The following section explains why motor skill practice should be a component of your routine and outlines how to structure its practice. Including motor skill practice adds variety and enhances engagement motivation, stimulates the central nervous system, mitigates our increasingly more virtual/less textural world, and leads to growing your activity repertoire and deepening your Iron Footprint.

For How It Adds Variety to Your FitBASE Routines:

Motor skill practice can be organized so its execution is sufficiently intense to qualify as a FitBASE component. For example, dribbling around obstacles can elevate heart rate into its training zone; the same is true with throwing and catching when running "routes" of a certain distance akin to a football receiver. The more options we have for engagement, the less likely our routines become stale and uninteresting.

For How It Affects the Central Nervous System Differently From FitBASE Engagement:

Motor skill practice affects the central nervous system unlike routine FitBASE engagement because its execution calls on different sensory information. Playing catch, kicking a ball toward a target, or dribbling a ball around obstacles demands cognitive and perceptual function. This stimulates growth to the cortical and subcortical regions of the brain that otherwise would not be triggered during FitBASE cardiovascular and weight training.

The learning (brain growth) that motor skill practice promotes can be especially important as we age. Independence can depend upon sustaining activity that requires multidimensional brain processing. In general, the more that sensory processing is stimulated, the greater the likelihood of preserving cognitive integrity.

For How It Can Mitigate the Contemporary Phenomenon of More Virtual/Less Textural:

Technology has rendered our lives more sedentary than ever, and more virtual/less textural. Cyberspace offers shopping, banking, business conduct, communication, *and* activity engagement. While saving gas preserves the environment and avoiding the frustration of lines at the store preserves our psyche, engaging in virtual activity seems like technology gone too far. Using your power to lift a piece of iron over your head is worlds different from swinging a joystick to activate an avatar to hit a golf ball, or programming data into a weight machine computer to establish the "level" of resistance.

Engagement needs texture to invoke our senses. Virtual engagement is pretend play or playing at playing, and it does not (generally) yield the same health protection. Motor skill practice is a multisensory, textural experience. We process as we move through space, or throw or catch a ball. Motor skill practice provides the textural, sensory stimulation that technological advances lessen, thus contributing to our well-being.

Note: This topic is presented in greater depth in *Technology, Apps, and Iron Footprint Fitness*, a White Paper download available at the Iron Footprint Fitness Academy on www.ironfootprintfitness.com.

For How It Can Enhance Your Physical Activity Repertoire:

Improved motor skill proficiency can broaden your activity repertoire. Sadly, many people do not develop competencies during their formative years, as the primary factors are practice opportunities and competent instruction. If you experienced quality physical education while in school, played sports, or otherwise engaged in backyard catch or similar activities, you probably can execute most skills in a proficient, purposeful manner. But your skills likely are underdeveloped if you did not have these opportunities, and the scope of activity you are able to engage in is comparatively limited, as you do not possess the proficiency to, for example, play softball or basketball. A limited activity repertoire (thin Iron Footprint) does not have to impact engagement motivation, but adherence is more likely with more choice, *and* you can gain additional health benefits by accumulating greater amounts of activity.

For How Growing Your Physical Activity Repertoire Can Enhance Your Engagement Motivation:

Motivation drives our decision to engage in activity, as well as how much effort we expend during engagement. We will engage if motivated, and the stronger our motivation, the greater our effort. While motivation is a complex concept of broad scope, self-efficacy—the belief we have in our ability to perform a task successfully—is especially applicable to this point. If we perceive that we can do a task, we will be motivated to do so. Past performance is the strongest determinant of self-efficacy. With previous success, the motivation to engage again is strong, but with limited past success, the motivation to engage again is weak. Self-efficacy is situation specific, so it can differ from one physical activity to the next.

With underdeveloped motor skills comes a limited activity reper-toire, for without feeling adequate to engage in an activity, you likely won't, nor will you venture into new activities, especially those out-side of the gym. This limits your engagement choice and discourages context-based engagement (e.g., sports leagues, pickup sports games), both of which can foul engagement motivation.

Choice is an exercise adherence principle. The more engagement options, the more you can refresh your routine. A routine dulled from repetition risks abandonment due to boredom. Possessing developed motor skills increases engagement options, for you will be confident in your adequacy to participate in many. On any given day, you can choose the most appealing engagement.

Similarly, while FitBASE activity is meaningful for certain reasons, engagement outside the gym is meaningful for others. Participating in sports has a different purpose from lifting weights at the gym. Applying motor skills within a context is an engagement purpose that cannot be fulfilled by completing a FitBASE routine, nor can the purpose of lifting weights be fulfilled by playing basketball. The greater your activ-ity repertoire, the more you can satisfy different types of engagement purpose.

Adding motor skill practice to your routine can boost engagement motivation by strengthening activity-specific self-efficacy, increasing engagement choices, and enabling engagement in activities with dif-ferent purposes from the gym. The practice will also create additional opportunity to track engagement achievement.

For How It Adds Novelty to Your Engagement Routine:

The novelty of motor skill practice can impact FitBASE motivation. Over time, routines can become monotonous, or too routine. While routines can yield health protection, novel activities—those new to the mix or infrequent enough that they seem new—are a welcome stimulus. They induce excitement, anticipation, and heightened attention, which stirs our motivation to do them. With motor skill practice, you get to move differently than usual, which offers

- new stimuli to pay attention to,
- another way to express your physical reality,
- another way to impress your Iron Footprint, and
- new scenery to look at, considering its practice will likely require using a different part of the gym than usual, or going outside.

FitBASE routines yield critical health protection, but the sameness of the routine can stagnate emotional engagement and plateau Iron Footprint growth. Adding motor skill practice shakes the "routine" out of the routine.

OK, I Get It and Commit to Adding Motor Skill Practice to My Routine!

How well do you throw? Catch? Kick? How adept are you at twisting and turning as you move? Ambling around obstacles? Going under and over obstacles?

Motor skill practice can enhance your FitBASE routine, stimulate your central nervous system, strengthen your engagement motivation, and grow your Iron Footprint. It can also be novel, fun, exciting, and a positive distraction.

Ask yourself the following questions to begin:

- *What motor skills do I practice, and how should I get started?*
- *How much time should I spend practicing motor skills?*
- *How often should I practice motor skills?*

What Motor Skills Do I Practice, and How Should I Get Started?

Three types of motor skills exist:

Locomotor skills are modes of movement:

crawling, walking, running, hopping, skipping, galloping, jumping
Non-locomotor skills qualify movement but do not produce movement:

twisting, turning, bending, rolling, stretching, balancing
Manipulative skills maneuver implements:

throwing, catching, striking (hitting), kicking, punting, dribbling

There are infinite possibilities about how to add motor skill practice to your routine and how to structure its practice. The following strategies can help you formulate a plan.
Suggestions for how to include *locomotor* and *non-locomotor* skill practice into your routine:

1. Select one locomotor skill and designate a straightaway approximately 20 yards long. Make sure it is free from debris, equipment, and at least the width of your arm span.

   a. Establish a time interval, e.g., 20 seconds, and move according to the selected mode from one end of the straightaway to the other, repeating the movement after 20 seconds have elapsed. With a set time interval, your rest depends upon how quickly you complete each length of the straightaway. For example, if you finish a length in 15 seconds, you can rest for five seconds before completing another length. You can adjust the time interval according to your heart rate. If your heart rate exceeds your target training zone, then increase the interval to provide more rest and reduce the intensity of your work. Conversely, if your heart rate is below your target training zone, then decrease the interval to increase the intensity of your work. Over time, it will take a shorter interval (more intensity) to prompt your heart rate into your target training zone. This is because your cardiovascular system has strengthened!

   b. Establish a certain amount of time, e.g., five minutes, and see how many laps you can complete in that time using the selected movement mode. Rest for two minutes, then repeat for a total of three to four times. Challenge yourself to complete more laps each set you do, but check your heart rate to ensure that you are maintaining your target training zone.

3. Use combinations of locomotor skills to complete the above sets. For example, skip one length and then hop back, or gallop one length and then run backwards the next. The combinations are endless, and for more variety (and novelty), add weight training. Complete one lap of the locomotor movement, then complete one set of eight repetitions using dumbbells. Sequence each major muscle for three sets: biceps, triceps, lats, pecs, deltoids, quads, hamstrings (or focus on one group).

4. Select one non-locomotor skill and add that skill to the execution of the above sets. For example, move in a zigzag pattern from one length to the other (regardless of the selected locomotor movement), and then return by moving in a spinning pattern.

5. Create an obstacle course that requires different types of locomotion, different qualities of movement (going under a barrier, going over a barrier, moving in straight and diagonal patterns), and different manipulative skills (moving and tossing a scarf/ball). The possibilities are endless!

Note: Depending upon the duration of this cardiovascular engagement (and number of weight-training sets), you may need additional activity so that your accumulation is sufficient toward inducing the health-related fitness of both components.

Suggestions for how to incorporate *manipulative* motor skill practice into your routine:

1. Select one manipulative skill and work on that skill through a practice progression—a series of increasingly difficult tasks related to the execution of a skill (refer to the end of this section

for practice progression outlines). Begin your practice with a task that matches your ability, and then work on more challenging tasks as your skill improves. Once you are consistently successful in executing a task, move to the next on the list, and so on. You will know when your performance is consistently successful. If not, work on the same task until it is.

A basic task progression for catching and throwing is as follows:

a. Toss a scarf into the air and catch it while standing.
b. Toss a beanbag into the air and catch it while standing.
c. Toss a whiffle ball into the air and catch it while standing.
d. Toss a scarf into the air and catch it while walking forward.
e. Toss a scarf into the air and catch it while walking backward.
f. Toss a beanbag to a partner and catch it from your partner while standing.
g. Toss a beanbag to a partner and catch it from your partner while shuffling sideways.

The written description of this engagement doesn't capture its potential for fun and excitement. Use ancillary means to create an environment that matches the fun. Music adds instant texture and is a positive distraction that sets an upbeat tone. If carefully selected, the tempo of your playlist can serve as a metronome for your intensity. Don't be surprised if others look to see what the commotion is all about. Help their Iron Footprints by inviting them to join!

How Much Time Should I Spend Practicing Motor Skills? How Often Should I Practice Motor Skills?

There is no guideline for how much time should be spent practicing motor skills (during one session or over the course of a week), or how often it should occur (each session? once or twice a week?). Two key considerations can determine the frequency and duration that makes sense for you: how quickly you hope to improve your skills (e.g., so you can play recreational basketball) and whether motor skill practice will occur during or separate from your FitBASE routine.

Motor-skill proficiency takes time and practice. If you intend to develop sufficient proficiency to engage in sports, and hope to do so sooner rather than later, then you need to commit to frequent practice of the longest duration possible—the more, and more often, you practice, the more quickly proficiency develops. If skill application is less urgent and practice will instead foster skills toward personal growth, frequency and duration are less critical. If this is the case, don't complicate the process by overthinking its inclusion—during one session add galloping and skipping, in another session add catching and throwing, and so on. Mix up what is included so you will reap the benefit of adding this component to your exercise routine.

If you are able to engage in motor skill practice *separate* from your FitBASE routine, then your schedule (frequency and duration of sessions) will be determined by how urgently you want to foster your skills. Since this engagement will occur separate from your FitBASE routine, you do not need to plan its infusion into your established routine.

Planning is required if your motor skill practice will occur *during* your FitBASE routine. The time you spend on practice during your routine depends upon the motor skill, engagement intensity, and the other physical activity that will occur during that session. For example, you could do locomotor skill work for the entire duration of your routine's cardiovascular component—if your engagement hits your target training zone—for each session of engagement. Considering the importance of variety to exercise adherence, engaging in motor skill practice as a cardio alternative is beneficial. But permanently replacing, say, the elliptical or treadmill with cardio-intense motor skill practice defeats the purpose. A mix of traditional and motor skill practice-based cardio will foster skill development and yield the benefit of variety.

You can also infuse weight training into your locomotor practice as a way of adding variety to your FitBASE weight-training routine. For example, after each completed episode of galloping or skipping, you could complete a set of dumbbell bicep curls (or targeting the appropriate muscle group for that session).

Motor Skill Practice Progressions

Motor skill proficiency is developed through practice, lots of practice. Even if you have the genetic capacity to throw a 100mph fastball, punt a football 60 yards, or kick a soccer ball so it curves at just the right moment to go into the goal from 30 yards away, you still have to practice these skills to fully develop your ability to execute them.

Motor skill practice though has to match your developmental level of performance to be especially effective toward fostering proficiency. This means doing activities that are neither too hard for you to successfully complete nor too easy that they don't challenge you to improve. Practicing a skill by doing an activity that is too hard will limit your improvement of that skill and risks eroding your motivation from frustration. Practicing by doing an activity that is too easy will stall your development and risks your motivation from boredom. If you are just learning how to throw, it will not serve you well to attempt to see how many times you can hit a small target from a distance because you likely will not be able to reach the target much less with accuracy. Maybe over (lots of) time and attempts you will ultimately hit the target, but it's more likely that your frustration will quickly dissuade you to continue. Likewise, if you practice a skill by repeatedly doing an activity that is too easy your ability will freeze at that level of proficiency. If you are learning how to kick a soccer ball into a goal and repeatedly practice kicking into the goal from two feet away this is the proficiency you will develop. Its application to the game of soccer is limiting but that may be a mute point if you lose your interest through boredom.

The answer?

Using a task (activity) progression to guide your skill practice can ensure that *how* you practice skills will most effectively aid your proficiency development. (*Note* – the term *proficiency* is meant inclusively, not to suggest that adding motor skill practice to your FitBASE routine is successful only if you develop exceptional skill abilities. The point is for you to develop your skills as fully as possible.)

Iron Footprint Fitness includes motor skill practice as a component of FitBASE engagement because proficiency is core to developing your physical activity self and is essential for immersion into context-based activities (e.g., sports leagues) that grow your Iron Footprint. It matters that you develop skill proficiency as best possible, so what follows are skill progressions to help you organize your skill practice and importantly help your practice be most appropriate to your (increasing) ability. In addition, a guideline is provided for how to create your own practice activities.

Progressive Practice Activities for Motor Skills

To use a progression, simply determine your point of entry and begin. If you are a beginner, know that you are low-skilled, or are not sure of your ability enter at level 1. You may have more proficiency than you realize and quickly move along the progression, or this may be just right. If you have played sports or otherwise know that you possess high skills, read through the progression to determine the entry spot that makes sense for you. Your sense of your physical self will inform your place along the continuum, and you will quickly know if your entry point is correct or needs adjustment.

How will I know when to move to a more difficult practice activity?

The rule of thumb is move to a more challenging practice activity when you can *successfully* execute the less-challenging skill activity *consistently*.

It will not serve your skill development to attempt to rush through a progression. It is not a race, although each progression you conquer is certainly a win! Consistent success means the VAST majority if the time you are able to complete the task. You will also know intuitively if your success is consistent or still random. 'Listen' to yourself as you practice to help determine when it's right to move to a more challenging task.

I have played sports all my life and consider myself high-skilled. Will / how can this work for me?

There is no end to a progression so even if you are already skill proficient there is always more challenge that can be created—you will not run out of runway. The 'formula' for how to do this is explained after the progressions are presented. Also, *The Motor Skill Coach* of the Iron Footprint Fitness Academy at ironfootprintfitness.com offers additional skill practice and progression information.

10-Step Motor Skill Practice Progressions

<u>Catching and Throwing</u>

While standing, toss a: scarf - bean-bag - nerf ball - beach ball - playground ball – yarn ball –softball - tennis ball – baseball – volleyball - basketball in the air and catch it (work the progression from scarf to basketball)

While standing, drop a ball and catch it on its return; let it bounce twice then catch it

With a partner, bounce pass back and forth while standing; while moving sideways

Throw a ball against a wall and catch it on one bounce; practice throwing to different levels

Throw a ball to a target on a wall; throw to targets at different levels

Throw a ball to a target (cone) while a partner defends the target

Throw a ball to a partner while they are moving

Throw a ball to a partner while both of you are moving

Throw a ball to a partner while avoiding a third person between you

Throw a ball to a partner while both of you are being defended

Challenges: throwing for distance, throwing for distance and accuracy, hitting a series of targets – 'spot throwing'- for time, play catch using baseball gloves, pitch off a pitcher's mound, throwing for speed, throwing different kinds of pitches (e.g., curveball, slider), catching at different levels

<u>Kicking</u>

Kick a stationary ball against a wall and trap it on its return

Kick a stationary ball against a wall using different parts of your foot and trap it on its return

(practice kicking to different levels of the wall)

Kick a stationary ball to a target on a wall and trap it on its return

While standing, kick a ball with a partner
Kick a ball to your partner while they are moving sideways
Receive a kicked ball from your partner while you move sideways
Kick with your partner while both of you move in different directions
Kick to your partner who is moving in different directions
Kick with your partner while both of you move in different directions
Kick a ball that your partner rolls to you from different locations

> Challenges: juggling, hitting targets of various sizes from various distances, kicking for distance, kicking for distance and accuracy, drop-kicking, scissor kicking, kicking off a tee

Dribbling (e.g., for soccer)

Dribble a ball through space while walking using the inside of your foot

Dribble a ball through space while walking using different parts of your feet

While walking, dribble to make shapes and along different paths (circles, squares; zig-zag, backwards)

Dribble in a straight line to a cone, turn around the cone then return to your starting point

Dribble around an obstacle course of objects while walking, then jogging

Dribble in a straight line while jogging, stop, control the ball then resume dribbling

Dribble as fast as you can around a cone and back without losing control of the ball

Dribble in a zig-zag pattern while jogging, stop, control the ball then resume dribbling

Dribble in space while your partner attempts to steal the ball

In a group of three, and inside a 20-ft radius circle, dribble while the other two attempt to steal the ball

> Challenges: dribbling around an obstacle course for time (while controlling ball),dribbling different-sized balls, dribbling around obstacles placed very close together, dribbling only with preferred or non-preferred foot.

Dribbling (e.g., for basketball)

Dribble a ball through space while walking; preferred and non-preferred hand

Dribble a ball around your body and through your legs while stationary; preferred and non-preferred hand

Dribble a ball through space using your preferred and non-preferred hand at different levels while walking

While walking, dribble to make shapes and along different paths (circles, triangles; backwards, spell out name)

While jogging, dribble around a cone and back; preferred and non-preferred hand

While jogging, dribble around a series of obstacles; preferred and non-preferred hand

Dribble around an obstacle course for time; preferred and non-preferred hand

Dribble in general space, stop, switch directions, stop, switch directions

Dribble in general space while your partner attempts to steal the ball

You and your partner dribble in general space and attempt to steal each other's ball

Challenges: dribble between legs (front to back and back to front) and behind back, preferred and non-preferred hand, dribble to a cone-sit down while still dribbling-stand up and return to starting point,

Punting (punting is a more complex skill than kicking so should follow kicking)

Strike a ball with your foot, preferred and non-preferred foot

Strike a ball with your knee, preferred and non-preferred foot

Strike a ball with your foot after it has bounced, preferred and non-preferred foot

Strike a ball with your knee after it has bounced, preferred and non-preferred foot

Strike a ball with your foot toward a target on a wall; practice to different levels, preferred and non-preferred foot

Strike a ball with your foot toward targets in general space (close and farther away), preferred and non-preferred foot

Strike a ball with your foot so it goes as high as possible, preferred and non-preferred foot

Strike a ball with your foot toward a target that is at an angle to your position, preferred and non-preferred foot

Strike a ball with your foot after an approach, preferred and non-preferred foot

Strike a ball with your foot after receiving a hike from your partner, preferred and non-preferred foot

Challenges: 'pooch' punting, punting while traveling (e.g., rugby)

Striking with a Racquet (e.g., tennis)

Strike a: balloon-yarn ball-racquet ball-tennis ball against a wall

Strike a suspended ball; suspend different sized balls from different heights

Strike a ball into general space for distance

Strike a ball to a target on a wall; practice at different levels and from different distances

Drop a ball then strike to different targets on a wall

Strike a ball overhead

Strike a ball to a wall consecutively

Strike a ball tossed by a partner

Strike a ball tossed away from you by partner

Strike a ball back and forth with a partner

Challenges: backhand striking, volley striking,

Striking with a Bat

Strike a stationary ball in general space

Strike a ball off a tee into general space

Strike a ball off a tee into general space

Strike a ball off a tee to different areas

Strike balls suspended at different heights

Strike a gently tossed ball

Strike a gently tossed ball to different areas

Strike a gently tossed ball to different levels and with varied force (pop-ups, grounders, line-drives)

Strike a self-tossed ball into general space
Strike a self-tossed ball toward targets placed at different levels

Challenges: preferred and non-preferred hand, hitting pitches from different angles, bunting

Striking with a Hockey Stick
Strike a stationary ball in general space
While walking in different directions, dribble a ball with a hockey stick
While walking, dribble a ball and start/stop and change directions and pathways on signal
While walking, dribble a ball in general space avoiding objects and other people
Strike (pass) a ball along the ground to a stationary partner
Strike (pass) a ball along the ground to a partner who is moving
Dribble and then strike (pass) a ball to a partner
Shoot a stationary ball (or puck) toward targets of different levels
Dribble toward a spot, stop, and then shoot toward targets of different levels
Receive a pass from a partner and then shoot toward targets of different levels

Challenges: 'spot-shot' shooting to specific spots of a goal (e.g., right top corner, left top corner, etc.), dribble ball or puck around body or behind back, wrist shots, slap shots

Volleying
Continuously strike a balloon upward while stationary
Continuously strike a balloon upward while traveling slowly in general space
(Repeat above using a lightweight ball)
'Set' a self-tossed ball overhead, then to a wall
'Pass' (forearm bump) a self-tossed ball to a wall
Underhand strike a ball back and forth across a low barrier with a partner
Receive a soft toss from a partner then set it overhead

Receive a soft toss from a partner then pass it back

Receive a soft toss from a partner then set it back to the partner who has moved locations

Receive a soft toss from a partner then pass it back to the partner who has moved locations

Set and pass different weighted ball back and forth across medium and high barriers with a partner

Challenges: volleyball serving,

Creating your own Motor Skill Practice Activities to Enhance your Proficiency and/or Sport-Specific Skill

Each progression described above is a basic outline of activities you can practice to foster your skill development. They also provide suggestions for activities you can do during the motor skill practice component of your FitBASE routine. Once you become familiar with these basics though you can use the information that follows to develop your own practice activities. This can be especially useful if you want to develop or improve your sport-specific performance. Designing your own practice activities takes but a bit of creativity, along with planning of course. You need to select the *skill* you are going to work on, the *equipment* you are going to use, the movement *pathway* you are going to move along (or have the equipment, e.g., ball, move along), and the *performance elements* you are going to work on.

1. Select the motor skill you are going to practice.

You may want to rotate among several different skills, or if you are interested in joining a sports league or improving your sports league play you can focus specifically on that sport's skills. To increase challenge, combine more than one skill. For example, practice catching while jumping, throwing while skipping, or volleying against the wall while traveling around the gym's perimeter. If you are high-skilled, practicing combinations offers unique challenge that is one way to continue to foster your proficiency. This type of practice may be unconventional but it can be very effective in helping you refine your execution. And, you never know when you will need to use skill combinations during sports play. If you dove to catch a fly ball during a baseball game then threw the ball to a base and got the base runner out who was attempting to advance you will be happy that you practiced throwing-after-sitting, or similar. Once you begin to brainstorm skill combination practice you will realize the possibilities are endless, and fun!

As a refresher, motor skills include the following movement patterns:
> *Locomotor skills* are modes of movement:
>> crawling, walking, running, hopping, skipping, galloping, jumping
>
> *Non-locomotor skills* qualify movement but do not produce movement:
>> twisting, turning, bending, rolling, stretching, balancing
>
> *Manipulative skills* maneuver implements:
>> throwing, catching, striking (hitting), kicking, punting, dribbling

2. Select the equipment that you are going to use.

Practice activities tend to be less challenging when using large, light-weight, slow-moving equipment, and more challenging when using small, heavy, fast-moving equipment. For example, lightweight and slow-moving throwing 'equipment' includes scarves, bean-bags, yarn balls, nerf balls, beach balls, and large whiffle balls. Heavy and fast-moving throwing 'equipment' includes baseballs, softballs, playground balls and footballs. If your goal is general skill development, then select equipment that best matches your level of performance. If your goal is to improve your ability to play a specific sport, then you may want to practice with the equipment specific to that sport, but keep in mind that different variations of equipment are available for most sports. 'Trainer' volleyballs are lighter and slower moving than regulation volleyballs, whiffle balls and plastic bats are lighter, slower moving and flight restricted compared to metal bats and baseballs, and cloth footballs are lighter and slower moving than regulation footballs. It is perfectly fine, in fact you should use the less-challenging equipment of a sport until you have developed the proficiency to use regulation equipment. This both helps your confidence and protects your motivation.

3. Select the movement pathway(s) you are going to move along or move equipment along.

Practice activities are less challenging when you are stationary, and more challenging when you are moving. As well, moving in certain patterns (pathways) tends to be more complex than moving in others. Catching and throwing to yourself while you are standing still is a less challenging practice activity than catching and throwing to yourself while you walk, which is a less challenging practice activity than catching and throwing to yourself while you move in a zig-zag pattern. Developing the proficiency to move equipment along different pathways is essential to many sports (e.g., controlling the hockey puck or soccer ball while you weave through the defense toward the goal), but enhancing your ability to move smoothly along different pathways is important to developing your physical self. (*Note* – please refer to p. 69 for a list of movement pathways – non-locomotor motor skills)

4. Select the element(s) of performance you are going to work on.

Practice activities are less challenging if you are simply attempting to execute the rudimentary movements of a skill (e.g., make contact with an object, or throw a ball into a general area), and more challenging the more precise you desire the execution (e.g., bunt down the third base line, kick a 30-yard field goal). If you are practicing a skill for the first time, or know that you possess limited capacity to execute a skill is, performance elements are secondary to becoming confident in its basic movement. For example, conquer successfully walking across a balance beam without falling before attempting to do so quickly, or in combination with other skills. If you are high-skilled and want to improve your sports league play then it is important that your practice activities emphasize the performance element(s) that will best increase your proficiency. Case in point, if you are a flag football receiver the more developed your ability to catch a ball away from your body the more likely you will help your team by being able to turn errant passes into completions. This means practicing making catches above your head, behind you, and side-to-side.

Other performance elements to practice include:
>Distance (e.g., kicking, throwing, punting)
>Accuracy (e.g., throwing or shooting to a target)
>Speed (e.g., foot speed and agility, throwing and kicking)
>Force (e.g., swinging a tennis racquet 'easy' for a drop shot)
>Executing a skill away from your body (e.g., hitting a tennis overhead)
>Directing equipment over or under a barrier (e.g., 'dinking' a volleyball,
>Reacting to equipment that is moving (e.g., fielding a ground ball, trapping a passed soccer ball, catching a rebound off a backboard)

Once you have established your skill focus, the equipment you are going to use, the pathway(s) you are going to focus upon and any specific performance element(s), you are ready to begin. Creating practice activities ought to be fun doesn't have to be daunting. The point is to use the suggestions presented to create practice that makes most sense for you and your ever-emerging proficiency. Some basic principles to keep in mind:

Less Challenging Practice:	More Challenging Practice:
Single skill practice	Skill combination practice
Lightweight equipment	Heavy equipment
Slow moving equipment	Fast moving equipment
Stationary practice	Practice while moving
Executing a skill without consideration for performance	Executing a skill specific to speed, accuracy, distance, etc.

For further information, please access the listed reference books. The first two listed present comprehensive, industry-leading knowledge about developing motor skill proficiency. The third listed presents information specific to exercise and sport psychology.

References

1. Graham, G., Holt-Hale, S. & Parker, M. (2012). *Children Moving: A Reflective Approach to Teaching Physical* Education (*9th ed*). McGraw-Hill Higher Education: New York, NY
2. Pangrazi, R. & Beighle, A. (2011). *Dynamic Physical Education for Elementary Students (17th ed).* Benjamin Cummins: New York: NY
3. Weinberg, R. & Gould, D. (2011) *Foundations of Sport and Exercise Psychology (5th ed)*. Human Kinetics: Champaign, IL

• • •

Notching FitBESTS: A 14-Day Start-Up Plan

FitBESTS are performance benchmarks (personal bests) of engagement "events"—physical activity trials within FitBASE and FitBUBBLE engagement.

Benchmark tracking is inherent to engagement because variables such as speed, distance, height, and weight can be objectively measured: How fast? How far? How many? How much? How high? Benchmarks are evidence of engagement achievement that is significant toward strengthening motivation, so the more achievement tracked, the better.

Conventional event trials (e.g., one-mile run, total sit-ups or push-ups) are familiar to many from competing in sports or taking school-based fitness tests, but FitBEST trials are to also include unconventional events that represent a wide range of engagement. Please review the FitBEST Trials Bank on page 36 for a list of suggested FitBEST trials.

Following are the principles that guide FitBEST imprinting, as well as a start-up plan to begin organizing your trials.

FitBASE FitBESTS Are Benchmarks of Your Gym Routine Engagement: Cardiovascular Strength, Muscular Strength and Endurance, and Flexibility

- FitBASE routines (daily workouts) must be intended to foster the health-related fitness components of cardiovascular strength, muscular strength and endurance, and flexibility. Track an equal number of FitBESTS for each component and sequence their trials. For example, on one FitBEST day, track a cardiovascular event; on the following FitBEST day, track a muscular endurance event, the next a muscular strength event, and the next a flexibility event. In addition, include motor- skill performance events in the FitBEST rotation following flexibility trials.
- The same or different events for each component can be tracked, but FitBEST trials for any one FitBASE event should be separated by two weeks. For example, do not repeat a June 1 push-up trial until June 14. Tracking the same events for a certain time cycle (e.g., four weeks) is the simplest start. New or additional events can be added after a completed cycle.
- Daily engagement is optimal, but complete at least four FitBASE workouts per week. The FitBEST start-up includes trials for each day of a four-day-a-week commitment. The number and frequency of weekly trials can be adjusted after completing the start-up.
- FitBASE FitBEST trials can occur during or after a workout. For example, a FitBEST one-mile treadmill walk time trial can frame that workout's cardio component, and a FitBEST muscular endurance trial of consecutive bench presses of a certain weight can frame that workout's weight-training component. FitBEST trials are purest when they occur after a workout, but time constraints may prevent this. If they occur during a workout, take care to ensure that the integrity of the workout is maintained. If a FitBEST cardiovascular trial only takes eight minutes to complete, you will need to do additional cardio exercise to comply with the engagement requirement to foster cardiovascular health.

- Be consistent in how you perform FitBASE FitBEST trials. You are the one cheated by inconsistency. Your health-related fitness is too important to compromise by inattention or sloppiness.

FitBUBBLE FitBESTS Are Benchmarks of Events That Occur Separate from Your Gym Routine

FitBUBBLE FitBEST trials can occur in *organized* or *unorganized* events. Organized events are put on for the purpose of drawing participants to the event. There is usually an entrance fee to participate, but this includes an event souvenir, typically a teeshirt. Unorganized events are those that you create and in which you are likely the sole participant. Iron Footprint Fitness advocates generous consideration for unorganized FitBUBBLE FitBESTS. The meaning of achievement and its impact on motivation is the same whether the benchmark occurs during sanctioned or unsanctioned events.

The most common *organized* FitBUBBLE FitBEST opportunities are endurance events such as running races, cycling races, triathlons/ biathlons, in-line skate races, "mud runs", and cross-country skiing races; or sport-specific competitions such as track meets, swim meets, or weight-lifting meets.

The first time you participate in organized events, it may be overwhelming—from parking to registering to getting to the start to doing the event—so allow plenty of time to arrive and get settled. For example, while at the starting line, look around, take a deep breath, and realize that *everyone* is feeling the same nervousness. Whether a novice or veteran, the dynamics of competition stir emotions each time the gun sounds. Experience may tame the emotion, but it won't go away. Nor do you want it to. The heat you feel fuels your effort to achieve new benchmarks. Welcome the heat!

While waiting for the event to begin, don't hesitate to strike up conversations with fellow participants. This will not bother anyone, really. And if you are brushed aside, what a jerk that person is! Chitchatting can calm your nerves, and you never know whom you might meet— perhaps a new workout friend, or more. As you continue to participate in organized events, you will begin to see familiar faces. This adds to the quality of the experience. Not only are you imprinting your Iron Footprint and notching FitBESTS, but you are also making social connections that you otherwise likely wouldn't.

After the event, note your time, imprint your Iron Footprint, notch your FitBEST if warranted, and then spend a few minutes at the post-event expo. This is usually located around the finish-line area and includes sponsor booths and tables. Food and water are also usually available. Water tends to be complimentary, and food sometimes is as well. The atmosphere of the finish area is powerful. There is a collective feeling of goodwill and accomplishment. Finishers readily trade "war stories" as they recount their experiences on the course. This is yet another social connection opportunity, and a chance to commit to (register for) your next event.

Last, observe the "24-hour rule" for wearing the participation or competition award you earned! Wear your medal proudly while you get groceries, pick up the kids, drop off the dry cleaning, and are at work the next day. Finishing medals are typically provided only for events that draw a large number of participants and/or cover distances no shorter than 10K (6.2 miles), but exceptions do occur.

For events that do not provide finishing medals, substitute the teeshirt to observe this important part of the experience. The 24-hour rule documents your achievement and generates acknowledgement from others. Nothing wrong with that! Humility is the rule, but fair is fair—the event was public so it's okay to publicly show the fruits of your labor.

Unorganized FitBUBBLE FitBEST events are limited only by your creativity. There is no right or wrong way to design them so long as your engagement is consistent for each trial of each unique event. For example, if you FitBEST a one-mile time trial on a track, you need to start and stop at the same place each time you do the trial, and start and stop your watch the same way from one trial to the next. If you have a background of physical activity-related competition, you likely can think of a number of events to begin to put to trial. If you don't have a competitive background, you may be challenged initially in creating events, but over time this will get easier. The FitBEST Trials Bank will help you start to generate ideas.

The following outlines a plan to help you begin to organize your FitBEST trials. Each event is described below.

14-Day FitBEST Start-Up

Sunday	Monday	Tuesday	Wednesday	Thursday	Friday	Saturday
	One-Mile Treadmill Walk for time		Total Push-ups		One-Repetition Max Bicep Curl*	Sit and Reach
Standing Broad Jump	Jump-Rope Revolutions in five minutes	Total Sit-ups		One-Repetition Max Bench Press*		One-Mile Time Trial on a running track or neighborhood course**

<u>One-Mile Treadmill Walk</u> (cardiovascular trial): At zero incline, and with arms swinging alongside your body, walk one mile on the treadmill as quickly as possible. Carefully increase the speed and maintain control over your feet. Immediately decrease the speed if you begin to lose your balance or reach for the handrails for support.

<u>Total Push-Ups</u> (muscular endurance trial): From either a regular or modified (on knees) position, and keeping your back straight and glutes and abs tight, lower yourself to a 45-degree elbow bend (about four inches from the ground, and then push up to the start position. Perform as many as possible until failure. Maintain a consistent tempo, not pausing at the top, one second down and one second up.

<u>One-Repetition Maximum (RM) Bicep Curl*</u> (muscular strength trial): Keeping your back, glutes, and elbows against a wall, curl a barbell from its resting position—along your upper thigh with your elbows straight, to its finish position—touching just below your shoulders. Do not use momentum to swing the barbell to its finish position. For your first trial, select a weight you know you can curl; carefully attempt more weight until failure to complete.

<u>Sit and Reach</u> (flexibility trial): Sitting on the floor with your legs straight in front of you, slowly lean/stretch forward from your pelvis as far as possible, reaching with your arms. Repeat three times, and use a body part to gaugethe farthest you reached forward—calf, ankle, past toes,

and so on. Reach forward slowly and in one motion. Avoid jerking forward or restarting your forward motion after a pause.

Standing Broad Jump (motor skill trial): Place your toes on a starting mark (masking tape, groove on floor) and jump forward as far as possible, keeping your legs together and landing on both legs simultaneously. Mark the spot of your rearmost heel. If you step backward, re-jump until the landing is held. Do three successful trials. Measure the farthest distance jumped.

Jump-Rope Revolutions (cardiovascular trial): Count the total number of jump-rope revolutions completed in five minutes using the jumping style of your choice, e.g., single jumps with feet together, single jumps alternating feet (skipping). Restart and resume counting from where you left off after a miss.

Total Sit-Ups (muscular endurance trial): Lying on a mat with knees bent at a45-degree angle, with someone holding your feet (or your feet carefully placed under a weight) and your arms crossed at your chest, curl up until the back of your arms touch your knees. Lower yourself to the starting position (shoulder blades touching the mat) and repeat. Maintain a consistent tempo, not resting at the top. Avoid starting and stopping. Continue until failure.

One-RM Bench Press* (muscular strength trial): Using a barbell and flat bench-press bench, and keeping your glutes, back, and head in contact with the bench, lower the barbell to your chest and press to the starting position without pausing (elbows nearly, but not quite, locked). For your first trial, select a weight you know you can press; carefully attempt more weight until failure. (Use a bench-press machine as an alternative to using a barbell and flat bench-press bench.)

One-Mile Time Trial** (cardiovascular trial): Complete one mile as fast as possible. Take care to note if the track is drawn in meters or yards so that your one-mile trial times are valid if you run them on different tracks.

*One-RM trials need to be *carefully and precisely* conducted. Seek assistance from a qualified fitness professional to master the movement before you attempt maximum lifts, and always use a spotter.
**If you do not have access to a running track, create your own "track" around your neighborhood or other safe location. Use the odometer on a car to measure one mile or close to one mile. No worries if you do not have access to an odometer! Simply decide upon a distance using the landmarks that are available. It could be from one house to another, or one store to another, or one tree to another. The creativity that can be employed to create events is the feature of unorganized FitBEST trials that make them so valuable to your development of resilient engagement motivation—there is virtually endless possibility as to the events you can create, and thus achievement you can track.

This start-up plan is an example of how to organize FitBEST trials. As you gain experience impressing this dimension of engagement, you will discover a trial cycle that fits best. Just as tracking benefits you, inviting your fellow engagers to do the same will add even more spice to this aspect of your routine. For example, you could designate one day a week or every other week as FitBEST day. You could also establish a friendly wager, with the spoils going to the one who shows the most improvement or completes the most of a specific exercise (e.g., push-ups, sit-ups, pull-ups, dips). Involving others adds another dimension of motivation, all the more stirring your adrenaline and driving achievement. You never know how you will inspire others, and others, you.

• • •

Embrace Competition

FitBESTS are performance benchmarks that invoke the spirit of competition, a notion that may stir discomfort and unease, even dread. Some of you may consider yourself 'noncompetitive,' and others of you may have had past humiliating competitive experiences. Indeed, but it bears to embrace for how it fosters achievement and nourishes engagement motivation.

Competition is a complex topic whose comprehensive description surpasses this essay. What follows considers its value to Iron Footprint engagement—it stirs adrenaline that sparks one's routine, and evokes new stimuli for sensory response.

Perhaps you had limited opportunity to compete in sports growing up, and it was painful. Maybe you only had limited instruction or practice before you were in a game overwhelmed, unable to make a positive contribution to the outcome. Or, your engagement was for public display, and your result felt humiliating. What many recall is performing fitness testing in school one at a time, in front of the class. Failing at the rope climb is one thing. Failing while the rest of the class looks on (and snickers, or worse) is another.

Public behavior, being compared to others, and a hyper-focus solely on the outcome are characteristics of competition that can invoke awful feelings. Being in a situation without adequate preparation to respond is painful, especially when it occurs in public theater. Physical activities that require you to engage at a performance level you are not capable of, and exaggerated notions about the outcome's significance foul its spirit. Competition itself should not be blamed for incompetent physical activity professionals who may have put you in a situation for which you were unprepared or placed way too much significance upon a game outcome. Rather, it ought to be embraced for how it inspires engagement FitBESTS by stirring energy that otherwise tends to be dormant during routine engagement.

Considering FitBESTS' significance to resilient motivation, competition adds value to engagement that trumps any lingering residue from past unpleasant experiences. However, just as it stirs adrenaline that pushes FitBESTS, it can also stir anxiety – competition can feel risky because you put yourself on the line toward an unpredictable outcome, and often do so in public theater. Whether pitted against your own FitBEST or others in organized events, what will transpire from start to finish is unknown. This dynamic can seem daunting because it is sharply contrasted to the predictability of FitBASE engagement—sometimes to the point of routines settling into a gym-induced monotonous trance— where there isn't the unknown to fear. Testing ourselves in competition deepens our Iron Footprint but the uncertainty, and the unknown can cause trepidation. Can I do this? How will I measure up? Am I going to finish dead last? Will I be disappointed?

There is too much to gain from competition to avoid it, and maintaining perspective can allay the unease. First, for conditioned or under-conditioned, experienced or novice competitors, the fear of coming in dead last can erode motivation to enter an organized race or similar activity. However, from one who has finished last in an organized running road race (then promptly vomiting into the weeds that lined the finish chute), I was not chastised by the other participants, and the sun rose the next day. Finishing last AND vomiting at the finish line. Ouch! But, so be it. Considered from the 'what do others think' standpoint nothing awful happened.

Another factor that can sabotage motivation to embrace competition is unease about 'putting ourselves on the line.' First, we are putting ourselves on the line—but for that particular event at that exact time, and a refreshing characteristic of engagement is the inherent opportunity for do-overs. So today you were 0-for-the-day batting (didn't get any hits), tomorrow brings the magic of a new game. Or, you finished dead last in a race and vomited at the finish. There is another scheduled for next weekend so a new chance to improve your finish and/or not get sick!

Second, in some capacity we put ourselves on the line at work and at home every day—different venues than competitive engagement, but similar dynamics for both present scenarios that require weighted decisions. The ones made at work perhaps impacting co-workers, your professional reputation and your work product itself, and those at home impacting the relationship you have with your kids and/or your partner. While your decisions can potentially put you at odds with your work or your family, you use your judgment to determine the best possible conclusions.

The sentiment is similar when you compete in activity. You put yourself on the line because the outcome *is* unpredictable. This means being vulnerable to disappointed results and/or comparisons to others, but the risk/reward overwhelmingly favors reward. Uncomfortable circumstances often stimulate growth. If we avoid 'putting ourselves out there' we miss opportunities to grow.

Embrace competition for how it can inspire your effort, grow your activity portfolio, and help you attain levels of performance otherwise unlikely. Your physical self will appreciate it!

• • •

The Change Process: Realistic Transformation

You decide to adopt Iron Footprint Fitness as your approach to activity engagement, are excited to create your achievement icon and watch your portfolio grow, and, heck, are excited to include motor skill practice into your routine even though you haven't dribbled a basketball in...decades. If you are like many of us, you are also anticipating how your new commitment to activity is going to impact your physique. Over time, and with consistent engagement of appropriate intensity, a degree of transformation can occur as well as improvement to aspects of our vascular and metabolic systems. Measures of blood pressure, blood sugar, resting heart rate, and cholesterol, along with others can pierce (more) deeply into that which is considered healthy, and losing weight, and/or increasing muscle mass will visibly change the shape and contour of our body. But a great degree of confounding and non-sensical misinformation exists about body transformation that can lead to expectations for radical change that are wholly unrealistic. This is critically problematic because the disappointment of not seeing the hoped-for, in some cases promised change, can erode motivation.

For example, not a novel claim, but as prevalent as ever and especially directed toward women, is the notion that exercise can spot reduce. This is an erroneous fallacy. It is impossible to lose size in one area of your body without losing size across your body. If more energy is expended than taken in we will lose weight, but size reduction is not spot specific. So-called trouble spots will transform along with the transformation that occurs across the body, but to a degree. Each of us bears a genetically determined number of adipose (fat) cells and distribution pattern amid our body. Diet and exercise won't eliminate adipose cells, but CAN REDUCE THEIR SIZE, and with it a change to our physique. But any change is across the body and any change specific to a body part is dependent upon our genetic makeup.

Another erroneous claim is that muscles can be lengthened (beyond what is anatomically possible) by engagement that promotes flexibility (yoga, pilates, stretching, etc.). Muscle fiber is plastic, like a rubber band that stretches then returns to its original length. Joint range of motion is largely determined by muscular suppleness so engagement that purposefully sustains plasticity will foster ease of movement. But since muscles attach to our skeleton at fixed points, lengthening, as it can be suggested, beyond the point of their attachment is impossible. Perhaps the claim is a phrase of semantics but taken at face value the expectation is grossly misleading for what is anatomically possible.

Also misrepresented is the degree to which our body's contour can change. Engagement that focuses on achievement-oriented health-related outcomes can change our body composition—less fat / more muscle—so a degree of welcomed transformation is possible. But as it can be implied, exercise cant entirely change the contour of what makes our body our body. For example, the ratio of our shoulder cage to our pelvis, or the ratio of our midsection to our legs, or that we were a 'square' at birth and continue to be a 'square' in middle age are physique variables predisposed by genetics. Regardless of how hard we try or what we have been led to believe it is unrealistic to think we can trump genetics through activity.

Hopefully these fallacies about exercise and body transformation seem ridiculous, but their persistence calls for continual redress and for addressing the realities of the change that can result from engagement. Managing our expectations about the transformation possible through engagement can mean the difference between sustaining or abandoning our routine. We will become discouraged if we seek unrealistic outcomes and either compromise our engagement or stop altogether. The first step in managing transformation expectations is considering 'change' from a fresh perspective.

Of the bodily transformation that engagement can foster, you:

> Will *feel a change before you see a change*
> Need to *prioritize how you feel rather than what you see*

Need to understand that *true transformation occurs from the inside out*

As a result of (achievement-oriented health-related) engagement, you WILL FEEL change to A) your emotional state, B) carrying out every-day tasks, and, C) participating in other forms of physical activity.

Each time you engage in activity you will likely feel its emotional impact. Engagement can induce the release of endorphins, so-called pleasure hormones, resulting in a 'runners high'. In addition, stress is relieved, and feelings of vibrancy, satisfaction, and self-pride are stoked.

Over time, often sooner than you may think, you also will notice how you feel stronger and/or more capable of completing common, everyday tasks. Cardiovascular capacity is strengthened from the first health-related engagement session and muscular capacity improves from the first occasion of resistance training (assuming engagement is with appropriate intensity). Muscles coming out of the gym are stronger than when going in (after regeneration), so it isn't long before you FEEL stronger while accomplishing common daily tasks. For example:

Carrying: a 1 gallon milk jug, case of water, case of soda, large box of laundry detergent, large bag of dog food, the vacuum cleaner up stairs, or a child—anywhere...FEELS EASIER

Walking: from the car to the office, the dog around the block, the dog at the park then throwing it a ball...FEELS EASIER

Changing: the bed sheets (lifting the mattress, tugging the sheets into place)...FEELS EASIER

Getting up: out of a chair, off the couch, out of bed, in and out of the car...FEELS EASIER

Putting on: nylons or socks while standing...FEELS EASIER

Reaching up: to get a coffee cup out of cupboard...FEELS EASIER

Noticing how: clothes feel (different) on (over time), and it FEELS like you control your body rather than your body controlling you.

Engagement will induce change that you first feel while going about tasks common to everyday life. It will feel easier to meet daily physical demands and you will do so with greater vigor. Engagement can similarly affect activities you pursue different from your FitBASE routine.

Whether league or recreational sports, or something else to impress a FitBUBBLE, your engagement in all forms of activity will feel different (good different), upon sustaining achievement-oriented engagement. Kicking or throwing a ball, shooting a basketball, controlling a golf club or hitting a forehand will feel different—easier, or that you have greater power or energy. The physical feeling aside, the sense of satisfaction or increased self-confidence that emerges is as powerful a variable toward fostering resilient motivation (recall how the attributes of hope and autonomy contribute to resiliency).

Approaching engagement as Iron Footprint Fitness enables you to capture your broadly considered achievement as a means to sustaining regular activity. This is a target-rich approach toward assessing your outcomes, a much more motivation friendly alternative than using (unrealistic) body transformation to drive your intent and determine your success. Realizing ALL your engagement success sustains your desire to continue, but recognizing the change in how you <u>feel</u> while going about daily life or engaging in activity may be the most important outcome, for how you feel is the first detectable change and perhaps the most significant.

To illustrate, in 2004, a reality TV show, The Swan, transformed so-called 'ugly ducklings' into proverbial swans. The process included extensive, usually full-body cosmetic surgery, makeovers, exercise sessions, and counseling to address emotional issues. Each week, two 'ugly ducklings' were pitted against each other to determine that week's swan. As part of the set-up, the participants were sequestered during their experience including not being able to see themselves until their dramatic reveal during an episode. All mirrors were removed from their sequestered residence, and care was taken to ensure they did not see themselves in reflections when traveling to appointments or while at the gym, the one I attended that was used for the exercise component of the transformation process—during taping all the gym mirrors were covered!

The participants began a standard exercise routine of cardio and weight training as soon as their surgeries healed. The gym was open to members during the time they trained, and overtime it became natural to exchange daily greetings. The show personnel dissuaded further interaction, but with no other segregation one couldn't help but overhear their conversations. The distaste of the show's premise and fact that these women seemed preyed upon aside (my opinion), it was fascinating to listen to their accounts of what they took away from each component of their transformation (surgery, makeovers, etc.). Many commented that exercise was the most 'real' component of the process. This seems to be a poignant example of how while engagement can change our body's look; its more powerful benefit may be how it makes us feel, both physically and emotionally. Through it we become able to navigate daily life vigorously (more so than if we do not sustain regular activity) and are emboldened with enhanced self-confidence.

The Swans didn't have the chance to feel the change that engagement can induce before their radical body transformation. Their bodies were invasively shaped and contoured and took on the appearance ideal that many seek from activity, yet according to an interpretation of their overheard comments, the outcome was hollow, if not meaningless. They looked different but didn't feel any different...

(Radical) body transformation is the variable we use most often to measure our engagement achievement for two reasons. We don't know differently and can fall prey to social notions about the ideal body. Success is transformation, anything less is failure. However, without invasive intervention, e.g., reconstructive surgery, the transformation we seek is wholly unrealistic, *and*, we feel changes before seeing them—we *feel* stronger before we see bigger muscles. Nevertheless, if we only know to look for changes (that we likely are not going to see), the ensuing disappointment erodes our motivation to engage until ultimately we stop even trying to try.

Iron Footprint Fitness offers a target-rich alternative that frames engagement as a multi-dimensional enterprise and allows for tracking achievement across all dimensions. 'Changes' are still felt before being seen, but the FitBASE, FitBUBBLES and FItBEST engagement you notch also creates a showcase of your achievement. You feel change but can also see your change via the growth of your portfolio.

• • •

Everyday Physical Activity Every Day

In the late 1960's while out for recess during elementary school, I would often see my mom jogging on the adjacent track in her heavyweight grey Sports and Health Club sweats and 'gym shoes'. My friends and I would wave. She would wave back then carry on with her jog, and we with playing the day's game.

My family valued physical activity. There was never a question of doing or not doing. We simply did, and it was simple to do. Convenient to access and nothing fancy. Catch in the backyard, games of starlight/moonlight in the empty lot, swinging on the swing set or climbing on its poles. There was no pretense to activity and merely opening the front door granted access. It was *everyday* physical activity, every day...

Everyday Physical Activity, Every day is an intentional play on words. Activity ought to occur every day, its access ought to be uncomplicated and its perfectly fine for it to be in something simple not fancy—like using the everyday plates rather than the good china, eating on the couch rather than in the dining room, or using paper rather than cloth napkins. There is certainly a time and place for the latter, but just as the world has profoundly evolved since the 60s, so too has the realm of physical activity. Sadly, engagement today can be anything but simple, convenient or accessible. Obvious barriers like space-limited built environments and the financial requirement to access certain types of activity exist. Perhaps less obvious, but equally constricting, perceived barriers also seem to exist from the undertones of how the now vast engagement industry markets and delivers activity. The following snapshots how obvious and less obvious barriers can make activity today anything but *everyday,* and be a formidable threat to its every day occurrence.

The majority of the US population lives in urban settings with limited green space. While some urban dwellers can afford to join exercise facilities, many are not able so have to exert energy to access suitable space before exerting energy being active. This can take its toll over time and ultimately dissuade engagement. Between a built environment that limits opportunity and no budget to join an exercise facility, many just surrender to the inaccessibility. But for those who are able to conquer access, other dynamics come into play that can equally risk 'every day' engagement.

Activity time for both youth and adults tends to be scheduled. Engagement doesn't just happen naturally as a part of one's day. Like going to the dentist, we make appointments. For some kids activity occurs only as scheduled by caregivers in the form of play-dates with other kids. If one hour is scheduled then one hour it is. Adults also carve out premeditated windows for engagement, but an interesting twist is that the activity form itself is dictated by when the engagement is scheduled to occur (e.g., I can go to the gym at 6 so I will take whatever group exercise class that is offered at that time). Perhaps this is an unavoidable circumstance of a frenetic paced world (and of course any activity is better than no activity!), but once engagement requires an appointment that dedicated time is its only allotted sliver. If the appointment is fulfilled, great, but an overbooked schedule hampers the agility required to reschedule if a complication interferes. A day of engagement is lost and with it, all the good that activity yields.

In this dynamic we seem to create a self-created access barrier. We limit our own accessibility by allotting only narrow, rigid windows of opportunity to engage. Perhaps it is an unavoidable circumstance of modern life that doesn't have an easy solve, but a barrier is a barrier. Then, for adults who belong to an exercise facility, engagement itself can be much less about *everyday* physical activity, particularly if the facility cultures more like a club than a gym.

Many exercise facilities are 'lifestyle centers' that partner spa-oriented services with fitness. These facilities tend to be beautifully appointed with contemporary flooring and countertops, and the latest generation of equipment set in areas with an armada of big-screen TVs that offer a menu of entertainment. Many also staff the floors with the directive to tend to members' needs, including wiping down equipment, re-racking weights and offering towels. At the risk of generalization, clubs purposefully frame members' engagement from the point of organizing one's belongings in the locker room to featuring branded workout attire at the gift shop to offering fresh-food post-workout replenishment. Gyms, comparably, house equipment and staff housekeeping to maintain a pleasant, functional environment. Members engage according to their own volition.

My experience actively belonging to (gorgeous) clubs and (functional) gyms simultaneously – no question, gym members sustain regular engagement much more so than club members do. While there is nothing inherently wrong with beautiful appointments; and who doesn't appreciate chilled eucalyptus towels, more engagement barriers can present in clubs than gyms.

Club members tend to approach their facility from a *"What can you do for me?"* perspective, with the 'do for me' less about health-related fitness than the ancillaries that are part of the club experience. Likely wholly unintended by the culture, club members seem to play **at** engagement more than really engage. Because there can be so much ancillary taken advantage of, actual engagement can become a watered-down version of what's necessary to elicit health protection. A little of this and a little of that can add up to a lot of nothing, fitness-wise (again, some activity is better than no activity). While engagement variety is an exercise adherence principle, at least the semblance of a program that appropriately impacts each health-related fitness component is needed. Flitting from one class to another, or a "Im going to do less cardio so I can sauna " or "I only have time for a few weights because I have a scheduled massage" pattern can form. A barrier to engagement can be the very environment and ancillary services that clubs proudly feature. Members' engagement can be sporadic and activities themselves can be seemingly fancy and whimsical, neither *everyday* physical activity, nor occurring every day.

(Gyms, comparatively, are approached from a *"How can I use you?"* perspective. With fewer ancillaries offered, engagement is the sole focus, and the engagement experience is about engagement. This creates a culture much more about *everyday* physical activity, every day.)

Further, under the mantle of 'Group Fitness', and regardless of the type of facility it occurs within, an ever growing array of classes are offered, including those that narrowly focus on specific body parts or particular components of fitness or forms of movement. For example, Ab or Glute classes focus on a segmented body part; flexibility, functional fitness, low-impact or Vo2 max classes focus on a particular component of fitness; and circuit training, Zumba dance, Belly dance and boot camp focus on specific forms of movement.

An ever-evolving menu of packaged activity offerings, including when and how often it occurs now dictates engagement for many. Exercisers narrowly frame their engagement around THEIR class and declare their activity identity accordingly; 'I do Pilates," "I do abs and glutes," "I do kick boxing." Related, the grey sweats worn universally to jog or play tennis or basketball have given way to activity- and climate-specific clothing and shoes from the burgeoning sports apparel industry. Just as engagement has become narrowly focused, clothes no longer multi-task. Cotton can certainly continue to be worn, but with high-tech fabrics that whisk perspiration, neutralize odor and all but do the engagement, the undercurrent of an established dress code has developed.

Rather than engaging in *everyday* physical activity, every day, access now is a package that specifies time, form and clothing – engagement occurs only as scheduled, then only in a narrow form of movement while wearing clothing that is specific to that form. While this does not have to resonate negatively, and while there is countless good about the growth of the fitness/sporting goods industry, an irony of the 'more' evolution is that it creates access barriers. Offering a greater variety, and more narrowly-focused engagement opportunities may have the opposite effect—offering more seems to result in less engagement!

Exercise facilities develop and deliver an evolving variety of classes to draw engagers. But statistics present a harsh counter. Our nation is more overweight and under active than ever. Nearly 60% of all adults carry excess weight and 2/3 fail to engage in the minimum recommended amount of activity to foster health protection, even while intending to. The fitness/sporting goods industry does not own these dismal statistics, but in the effort to increase membership by offering an evolution of narrowly focused, specialty classes it appears the public's interpretation has prompted engagement exclusion rather than engagement inclusion. It seems messages that emanate from 'packaged engagement' have created access barriers and the culture itself risks engagement motivation.

First, with packaging comes its marketing. Glossy print media depicts 'exercisers' engaged in the forms of activity (group fitness classes) offered. The sarcasm is because campaigns tend to use 'fitness' models to represent the clientele, but most fitness models are models wearing fitness clothes, photographed in ideal lighting with flawless hair and make-up, the final product air-brushed to minimize imperfections. Pretty faces and pretty pictures are to be appreciated but not when they cause a perceived access barrier. The *everyday* exerciser looks nothing like the depicted exerciser, significant because engagement motivation is strengthened by seeing another with whom we can identify engaging. We are much less likely to be enticed if it appears we are different than the others. Related, the depicted exerciser may also skew one's sense of exercise outcomes, for the one pictured is perceived to exemplify the appearance ideal we are to aspire to achieve. But, I can no more look like a leggy blond than a leggy blond can look like a stubby brunette. False hopes and unattainable expectations will only yield disappointment and erode engagement motivation.

Second, the evolution has prompted an interpretation that exercise specialists rather than exercise generalists are preferred. With packaged physical activity comes defining one's engagement according to the package selected. "I do yoga." "I do cardio." "I do boot camp." Once one declares to be a particular type of exerciser there is minimal motivation (or encouragement) to engage in other forms of activity, or even consider the need to do so. This interpretation can ding engagement motivation for two reasons—specialized, narrow engagement will elicit only limited outcomes, and engagement variety is a strong determinant of exercise adherence.

Then there is the circumstance when class is cancelled, or one's schedule is not amenable to the class schedule. Then what? Most likely NO engagement; for a specialist, unlike a generalist, doesn't possess the content knowledge to know what else to do. Case in point. Recently my gym had a brief but total power outage. As the group fitness class exited the studio some quickly found an empty stationary bike and resumed the semblance of a cardio workout. Most though emerged bewildered, scanned the cardio and weight equipment but stopped before advancing any further. Unclear how to resolve their dilemma they left, and when the power restored the group class resumed at a quarter of the participation. While there could have been a myriad of contingencies that prompted the others to leave, the clear disorientation, the sheer "I don't know what to do now" seemed the likely culprit.

The emergence of exercise specialists has also born a sub-population that approaches engagement from an even more micro focus—those who prioritize classes that focus on specific, segmented body parts. Ab classes, Glute classes or similar can accent a routine that addresses comprehensive health-related fitness, but engaged as stand-alones will not yield the intended results. One, spot reduction doesn't work. Two, engagement that only involves certain body parts will not induce the same level of health-protection as engagement that is full-bodied. Three, we are of one body and engagement ought to enhance the relationship we have with our body. Most classes that focus on segmented body parts do so from a deficit model – something has to be fixed. Working on our physical limitations as part of a full-bodied routine can engender our relationship with our physical self but targeting parts for their imperfection puts us at odds with ourselves. Related, if we only focus on what is 'wrong,' we miss the opportunity to foster our physical activity strength(s). Growing our Iron footprint by imprinting FitBUBBLES with all we do in engagement aids our motivation but it would be a shame to miss cultivating that which is a particular strength, for this also furthers the relationship we have with our physical self. An approach to engagement that isolates specific body parts is unlikely to sustain motivation. The hoped-for outcomes, which are unrealistic to begin with, are a set up for disappointment and its partner, motivation erosion. Full-bodied engagement has to balance segmented body part engagement.

Second, one might hesitate to participate in an activity for which one doesn't have its specific clothing. "I don't have yoga pants so I'm not going to go to yoga class." The hesitation may be short-lived realizing that soccer shorts are perfectly suitable for yoga class, but the perceived lack of activity-appropriate clothing may be reason enough to self-limit engagement in the activity. Interpreting engagement to require adherence to a dress code adds an unfortunate access barrier.

Especially unfortunate is that those who are under-active, and/or new to engagement (the 2/3 of the US adult population that fails to accumulate the minimum amount of engagement to yield health protection) are especially vulnerable to access barriers that have emerged in the evolution of the industry's growth and programming. Those inexperienced do not possess the capacity to discern engagement appropriateness – 'if the gym offers Abs class then that must be all I need," or realize the universal functionality of 'everyday' activity clothes. Those who are experienced or able to sustain regular activity may not realize that the hesitation caused by wondering about clothing can be enough pause to dissuade engagement. If this population does begin to engage in the segmented body part offering of the gym it's likely the outcomes yielded will mirror the limited scope of engagement which will threaten their already fragile motivation until sooner than later, they quit.

Exercise facilities offer more, and a greater variety of engagement opportunities than ever. But ironically, accessibility is challenged by the interpretation of this evolution and more has become less. It's time to return to the ideal of jogging around the school track in grey sweats and gym shoes – to approach engagement from the perspective of *everyday* physical activity, every day.

Access to engagement ought to be simple and uncomplicated, and its occurrence ought to be every day. If we have to dress up to engage, then only do it at its appointed time in its specified space and only focused on a segmented body part engagement becomes more about the process required to engage than the process of engagement itself. Formality is an unnecessary burden that is also ironic. While much of our lifestyle has become less formal, activity engagement has become more formal.

The world may no longer allow for the now sentimental notion of jogging around the neighborhood school's track, but the notion's ideal is the important recapture. Iron Footprint Fitness purposes an all-access, uncomplicated, simple approach to engagement and offers the means to organize daily activity and showcase the resulting achievement. Gym-goers and non gym-goers alike can use the approach to avoid or solve access barriers. As well, Iron Footprint Fitness also eliminates any 'rules' for engagement (beyond following the principles for yielding health-protection).

My current activity hero is a woman in her (estimated) late 70's who takes daily walks around the neighborhood in her comfortable sandals while holding her purse. What makes her engagement stand out is she purposefully climbs the sets of stairs leading to the townhomes that line the neighborhood, while doing bicep curls with her purse. Then, at the top of each set of stairs, she does knee bends with her purse held in front for balance, and at the bottom of each set of stairs, she stretches a body part, switching to a different body part at the next stairwell. Then, she checks her pulse after each stairwell's combination. We speak different languages but I wave at her and she waves back, I also give her thumbs-up, which she returns. This is the essence of Iron

Footprint Fitness--simple, uncomplicated yet purposeful engagement. It's *everyday* physical activity, every day!

. . .

Iron Footprint Fitness for Non-Gym Members and Home Gym Users

Many people exercise without belonging to a gym, and others mix gym membership with home equipment. Attaining health protection from engagement is not venue dependent, and one can impress their Iron Footprint just as well belonging or not to a gym. However, unique motivation challenges can exist for non-gym members.

Exercising at home can save time, gas and money and allow for engagement not tied to a gym's schedule. A common sentiment is that with availability and convenience, the motivation to exercise naturally follows. True, availability can positively influence motivation, but it alone does not guarantee consistent engagement motivation. Exercising at home means contending with distractions not present at the gym—and at the same time not having the benefit of tapping into distractions present in the gym environment.

At the same time, there is every distraction and no distraction

Exercising at home means the potential for being distracted by all that constitutes HOME. Children, pets, the computer, the phone, laundry are possible engagement interrupters, along with the compulsion to order the environment before or during engagement — we tidy up or clean. Of course, engagement can occur while the kids are at school, with the computer and phone off and after the dishes are done, but the temptation can persist to check email, send one more text and straighten up the room. Before long, distractions eat the time carved out to exercise.

Then,
At the same time, there is no distraction and every distraction

Exercising at home is an individual sport. We are alone with our thoughts as we follow the exercise DVD or otherwise push through cardio and strength training. The TV or radio can provide company but there is no chit-chat or camaraderie with fellow exercisers, no listening to the re-mixed playlist coming from the spinning class, no spying on the cute boy/girl, no watching the trainers for pointers or ideas about new moves, no looking for what the strange person is wearing today, no eves dropping on conversations, and most impactful, no drawing engagement inspiration from those around us.

While many home gym-ers mitigate the distractions (and lack thereof) and sustain regular exercise, others are challenged by what the home gym lacks – an exercise- dedicated built environment and the engagement motivation inspired by fellow exercisers.

Our home may be perfectly suitable for exercise but its configuration is obviously more amenable to sleeping, eating, relaxing, and socializing. Many CAN exercise in their bedrooms, dens, family rooms, or basements but others struggle to separate form and function. Traveling to the gym might be unpleasant but once there we operate with purpose and focus. 'Traveling' to the den to exercise to the DVD may be convenient, but once there it can be easy to become distracted.

Related, a powerful source of engagement motivation is the inspiration we draw from seeing others engage, especially those who we identify as looking/ similar to ourselves. Home exercisers cannot access this source of motivation, and if engagement is to a commercially-prepared DVD those featured tend to be uber fit, likely bearing little fitness-resemblance. This may not be noticed unless brought to our attention, but its reality isn't lost on our psyche. Ultimately, the disconnect weighs motivation.

A solve for home gym-ers who struggle to sustain regular exercise?

Approaching engagement as Iron Footprint Fitness can 'build the environment' that strengthens motivation. First, it offers a framework to organize meaningful engagement. Structuring each session according to FitBASE, FitBUBBLES, or FitBESTS enhances purpose whether following a commercially-produced exercise program or your own routine. Engaging with a clear purpose means our focus is more apt to be sustained than if we approach a session from a 'just' perspective, as in *I'm just going to do some cardio.'* The focus that is provided by engaging toward impressing FitBASE, FitBUBBLES or FitBESTS can help counter the loneliness that may arise when exercising solo.

Second, the intentionality of impressing your Iron Footprint influences the effort of your engagement. Engaging with optimal effort helps evoke achievement that nourishes your motivation for subsequent engagement, and feeds the cycle of sustaining (appropriately) intense engagement. This might be especially valuable to home-exercisers because they are not able to draw inspiration from being alongside others as they exercise and their intensity may slip because the social dynamic of 'working hard because I'm being watched' isn't relevant. FitBEST event trials can add accountability to engagement even when no one else is watching.

Third, actively impressing FitBUBBLES means growth to your activity repertoire and novel activities included into your routine. The greater your activity spectrum the more engagement choice you have on any given day, and variety lessens the likelihood of your routine becoming monotonous. Home exercise is ripe for monotony due to the routine of exercising alone to the same program in the same room. Actively adding FitBUBBLES to your Iron Footprint can counter the routine of the routine by its byproduct of adding novel activities to your day-to-day engagement as well as growing your portfolio from which you can exercise (no pun intended) daily engagement choice.

Engagement motivation for those who home-gym can be differently challenged than for those who go to a gym. Approaching engagement as Iron Footprint Fitness counters the negative distractions that can be present when exercising at home, and can be a substitute to the positive distractions present at the gym but not present at home.

Summary and a Peek Ahead

The Iron Footprint Fitness approach to physical activity is unique to the field for its purpose, content and agility. It offers a solution to inconsistent motivation by framing engagement as a multi-dimensional enterprise, outlining the generous opportunity for achievement that exists across the dimensions and presenting how showcasing achievement can foster resilient motivation to sustain regular activity; introduces motor skill practice as a recommended component of FitBASE engagement; explains the importance of FitBASE engagement being *Achievement-Oriented Health-Related*; and is aligned to the principals known to increase the likelihood of adherence to an activity program.

It is also free of cost to adopt, easy to adopt, and can be used by anyone regardless of age, gender, previous activity history, level of skill or performance proficiency, or whether they belong to a gym or are a home-exerciser. At the same time it can (re) introduce disgruntled or frustrated exercisers to an activity approach that is user-friendly, it can also inspire high-skilled activity veterans to hit new performance benchmarks.

Part V describes how to take the important, meaningful and inspiring next step of creating and beginning to imprint your Iron Footprint icon. It also outlines the features of ironfootprintfitness.com that you can access through the membership granted by purchasing this book.

NEXT STEP – BEGIN TO IMPRINT YOUT IRON FOOTPRINT TODAY: SELF-CREATE OR ACCESS THE PLATFORM AT THEIRONFOOTPRINTFITNESS.COM ONLINE COMMUNITY, THE PAVILION

Today is the day, rather *now* is the time to begin to imprint your Iron Footprint. You can either create your own achievement icon or use the platform provided on www.ironfootprintfitness.com.

If you are going to create your own icon, brainstorm to decide the marks, symbols, and diagram you are going to use to depict your FitBASE, FitBESTS, and FitBUBBLES. Review the suggested protocol for how and what to consider as achievement within each dimension; then put pen to paper and start to reap the motivational benefit of seeing your accomplishment. Don't over think the process or get mired by attempting to create a perfect icon. It is absolutely ok for you to adjust your icon's shape or form as the imprinting process takes hold, in fact this is likely once you begin to see your Iron Footprint grow and realize different ways to refine its display. You can also use the example templates provided in the Appendices to help you get started.

Iron Footprint Fitness Online

Otherwise, activate your complimentary membership to ironfootprint-fitness.com to access numerous assets to grow your iron footprint and foster resilient motivation including, *The Pavilion*, the Iron Footprint Fitness member's community. Along with other features, *The Pavilion* offers a social platform to compile your Iron Footprint, report significant FitBASE, FitBEST and FItBUBBLE achievement for community recognition and connect with fellow members. In addition, the website also includes a trainer-locator you can use to find a physical activity professional (e.g., personal trainer) who delivers physical activity as Iron Footprint Fitness. Trainers can provide priceless support. Better yet is one who can support your Iron Footprint Fitness approach to engagement.

Please read below for further description of the website's available resources. To create your account, please go to the registration center on the Homepage then enter access name: achievement and access password: motivation at checkout.

From there you will enter *The Pavilion* where you can:

- Use the platform to create your Iron Footprint
- Join a special-interest community
- Submit your significant achievements for FitBRAG recognition
- Access 'Barriers-Solutions' to enlist help to overcome an engagement challenge or offer a solution to another member's challenge
- Download *Certified or CertiFRAUD? Assessing the Professional Competency of Your Personal Trainer – Who's Minding Your Store?* to aid your selection of a personal trainer or ensure the professional competency of your existing trainer.
- Access 'Tools and Tips' including, exercise tips, activity planning templates, motor skill practice suggestions

- Download special topic White Papers including (some that you have already read in Part IV):
  - KidPRINT
  - Women and Iron Footprint Fitness
  - Embrace Competition
  - Senior Adults and Iron Footprint Fitness
  - Exercise Adherence and Iron Footprint Fitness
  - The Change Process
  - The Power of "ER"
  - Everyday Physical Activity, Every Day
  - Technology and the "Hasn't-Done-It" Generation
  - SportPRINTS/TeamPRINTS
  - Achievement-Oriented, Health-Related Fitness
  - Motor Skills
  - 14-Day FitBEST Start-Up Plan
  - Iron Footprint Fitness and Home-Gym Users
  - 30 BEST Days

A quick note about this seemingly random buffet of topics:

Iron Footprint Fitness can be adopted universally, as the approach is neutral to gender, age, ethnicity, culture, and sport preference, etc., but characteristics specific to certain groups can present unique engagement dynamics that bear attention.

Knowledge is power, and the more you know about what might uniquely influence your engagement, the better prepared you will be to mitigate challenges. You may see yourself in the special topics or not. Regardless, they present additional information from which to consider engagement and achievement. New White Papers will be added to the library on a regular basis. It is anticipated that feedback from the community will generate topics as well as those delivered by Iron Footprint Fitness.

Summary

Whether self-created or by accessing the platform on ironfootprint-fitness.com, begin today, better yet, begin now, to showcase your physical activity achievement. You deserve the boost it can inspire!

FINAL THOUGHTS

Sustaining regular physical activity can be a challenge, even for the most motivated. But sustain we must, for nothing else has the same impact on our well-being.

Sadly, many of you have suffered through engagement due to more reasons than can be detailed here, and are haunted by painful memories of humiliation. Your subsequent lack of interest is understandable, but risky. Others of you have endured less egregious indignities, but still struggle with engagement motivation, as well as sustaining a routine that yields optimum benefit. Then there are those of you who manage to get to the gym more often than not, but contend with phases of uncertainty and uninspired effort due to hitting performance plateaus.

Circumstance aside, discouragement from the perception that you are not achieving (even when the desired achievement is unrealistic to begin with) is the culprit. Discouragement brings out the grumbling gremlins that erode motivation until the flame that fuels engagement's drive is finally suffocated, along with the health protection yielded. But there is hope!

Iron Footprint Fitness supports engagement motivation by transforming the notion of physical activity achievement. As a multidimensional enterprise, engagement achievement can be tracked for how it occurs across each dimension. Different from the dangerously narrow view that typically gauges success, Iron Footprint Fitness outlines engagement's generous potential for achievement, and offers the means to capture it for display.

As mentioned earlier, Iron Footprint Fitness isn't a gimmick or a miracle. It doesn't take the necessity of exertion away, but it does ease the effort required to get to the gym or go for a run or play basketball at the park. It nourishes and protects your motivation to engage today, and then again tomorrow and the days after tomorrow.

And it drives the grumbling gremlins away.

Smile while you attempt to beat your push-up benchmark, take your place in a new group fitness class, count jump-rope revolutions, practice free throws...SMILE.

APPENDIX A: QUICK REFERENCE DEFINITIONS AND FREQUENTLY ASKED QUESTIONS

Definitions

Iron Footprint - a graphic portfolio of physical activity achievement according to daily routine engagement (FitBASE), performance benchmarks (FitBESTS), and the different types of physical activity engaged in (FitBUBBLES)

Iron Footprint Fitness – an approach to physical activity that fosters resilient motivation by framing engagement and recognizing achievement according to the dimensions of FitBASE, FitBESTS and FitBUBBLES

Iron Footprint Portfolio – a compilation of physical activity experiences according to theengagement dimensions of FitBASE, FitBESTS and FitBUBBLES

Resilient Engagement Motivation / Engagement-Resilient Motivation – a consistent desire toengage in physical activity driven by the hope and autonomy that is fostered by showcasing FitBASE, FitBEST and FitBUBBLE achievement in an Iron Footprint

Achievement-oriented, health-related workout – physical activity engagement in cardiovascular exercise, weight training and stretching according to the intensity required to build cardiovascular and muscular capacity and improve flexibility

FitBASE – a measure of physical activity achievement that recognizes the completion of an achievement-oriented health-related workout

FitBUBBLE – a measure of physical activity achievement that recognizes activity done separate from or in addition to a FitBASE workout, and each different type of activity experienced

FitBEST – a measure of physical activity achievement that recognizes a personal performance benchmark

The Pavilion – the ironfootprintfitness.com portal for members to create and maintain their Iron Footprint pages; join special interest groups; access special topics downloads, physical activity resources, tips and tools; and access The Podium for member recognition, weekly challenges and member-contributed solutions to engagement barriers.

Iron Footprint Fitness Academy – the ironfootprintfitness.com portal that provides members with special topic resources to support their effort to sustain physical activity as Iron Footprint Fitness

• • •

Frequently Asked Questions

Why 'Iron' Fitness Footprint – what does the word Iron signify?

Good question! 'Iron' is a time-tested word synonymous to exercise and physical activity – it is of iron (or a contemporary amalgam) that most equipment used to enhance physical wellness is made; it's with many irons-in-the-fire that we want to approach engagement; and it's with an iron fortitude that we want to sustain regular engagement.

I purchased the book Iron Footprint Fitness. How do I access the membership features of the website?

First, thanks for purchasing the book! The book and the website are designed to complement each other so as an added value to the book's purchase you also have complimentary Membership access to the website. Complete Membership Registration on the website and at checkout enter access name: achievement and access password: motivation. This will create your complimentary user account.

I work with a trainer, can I still use IFF?

Yes. IFF is a perfect complement to working with a personal trainer. It doesn't supplant the important role of your trainer, but can help to ensure that your engagement is intentional, purposeful, meaningful AND achievement-oriented. You and your trainer can work together to devise a plan for motor skill practice and how to become immersed in community and context-based activities. And, of course track your achievement by imprinting your Iron Footprint.

How can I locate a trainer who follows IFF?

Simply use the trainer locator data base to access an IFF trainer suitable to you. (*note* – the selection of a trainer should be thoughtful, thorough and intentional. After all, it's your health and well being that your trainer is helping to foster. *Certified or CertiFRAUD? Assessing the Professional Competency of Your Personal Trainer – Who's Minding Your Store?* presents a two-step protocol to use to select a personal trainer or determine the professional competency of your existing trainer. It is available as a download at the Iron Footprint Fitness Academy of ironfootprintfitness.com. It can also be accessed at http://www.amazon.com/s/ref=nb_sb_noss?url=search-alias=stripbooks&field-keywords=certified+or+certifraud+assessing

I exercise to a video or follow a commercial exercise program, can I still use IFF?

Yes. Each component of IFF can be adapted to any exercise program. You can track your FitBASE, FitBESTS, and FitBUBBLES according to how each aligns to the program you follow. In The Pavilion of ironfootprintfitness.com you can likely find suggestions for how to compliment the program you follow with IFF. Chances are other IFF members follow the same program and may be able to provide ideas about how to organize your FitBASE, FitBESTS and FitBUBBLES.

Im new to exercise, can I use IFF?

Yes. Tracking your engagement achievement will help you develop resilient motivation regardless of your current pattern of engagement or level of fitness/performance. It will help you establish a consistent habit from the beginning. It will also inspire you to engage in other forms of physical activity besides formal exercise. This will grow your physical activity portfolio (the deeper and denser your Iron Footprint the better) and develop your physical activity personality.

I don't like to compete and I have never thought of myself as competitive. Why does IFF include competition?

IFF encourages competition because it stirs adrenaline which stimulates optimum effort which leads to personal performance benchmarks – an absolute marker of achievement! While IFF encourages competition against others, self-competition to improve FitBESTS has the same positive impact on motivation. Don't let poor past competitive experiences sour your consideration for new ones. IFF members can download a white paper on competition at the IFF Academy of ironfootprintfitness.com. This offers additional perspective on why competition can be so useful (and fun).

Im a senior adult, can I use IFF?

Yes. Tracking your engagement achievement will help you develop resilient motivation regardless of your age—even if you are a senior engaging in physical activity for the first time in your life! IFF members can download a white paper, *Senior Adults and Iron Footprint Fitness,* at the IFF Academy of ironfootprintfitness.com.

Can my kids use IFF?

Yes. IFF can have the same impact on motivation for kids as for adults, with some developmental modification to the focus of FitBASE, FitBESTS, and FitBUBBLES. IFF members can download a white paper, *KidPRINT,* at the IFF Academy of ironfootprintfitness.com for more information on how you can help your kids, or kids you know, develop an engagement habit that will last a lifetime. (As stated in our Terms and Conditions, kids under the age of 13 are not allowed on-line access, thank you.)

I exercise consistently and my motivation is strong, how can IFF help me?

The more achievement you identify the more you will want to identify—success begets success. IFF can help you define and realize achievement more broadly than how you have considered it, which will further develop your physical activity portfolio. Remember, your Iron Footprint ought to be as deep and dense as possible! IFF can also help you sustain an appropriate level of effort so you avoid hitting performance plateaus.

I really don't like to be active, how can IFF help me?

A lack of motivation to engage in activity is often because past experience has been unsuccessful – failing at gym class, missing the ball and getting hit in the face - most of us avoid what we don't feel we are competent to do. We also carry very narrow views about what achievement in physical activity is which limits the chance that success will be realized. IFF shows you how to broadly identify physical activity achievement and showcase it so you can 'see' your gains. Once you start seeing your achievement you will be motivated to achieve more. Success begets success!!

I'm a physical activity professional, what benefit is IFF to me?

IFF provides unique benefit to professionals from all corners of the physical activity industry, including; personal trainers, gym owners/ managers, fitness managers, coaches, youth physical activity program leaders (e.g., After-school, YMCA, Boys and Girls Clubs) youth group leaders (e.g., Boy Scouts, Girl Scouts, church groups), physical education teachers, recreation leaders, grant writers, community-based adult sport/activity clubs, commercial exercise program developers, and senior center program specialists. Examples of benefit include:

increasing your income by attracting more clients with your proven ability to yield results, sustaining a positive reputation as a program/gym that works, improving the attendance (and sustained registration) of members/participants, and using the approach to brand your programming. Please see *It Has...Value to Physical Activity Industry Professionals* located in Appendix C of *Iron Footprint Fitness* or on the homepage of ironfootprintfitness.com for more information about its value to professionals of the activity industry.

I'm a physical activity professional, how can I attract clients who want to follow IFF?

Simply pay a one-time fee of $25 to register on the *Iron Footprint Fitness Professional Registry*, located on the homepage of ironfootprintfitness.com

I can't afford to join a gym, and live in a small apartment in an urban area. Is IFF realistic for me to use?

YES! IFF can help you create a daily workout that will yield health benefits (review *Achievement Oriented Health-Related Fitness* in Part IV of this book or as a White Paper on ironfootprintfitness.com) using what is available to you (e.g., climbing a stairwell for cardiovascular exercise, doing push-ups to develop strength, using homemade weights for strength training). It can also inspire you to think of aligned, realistic FitBEST trials (e.g., how many times can you walk/run around your block in 20 minutes, how fast can you walk/run around your block once, how many squats can you do getting off your couch or chair in one minute, how many sit-ups can you do in one minute where you also (softly) toss a soft ball against the wall as you rise up (to practice the motor skill of catching) (old socks or rags can be balled up and taped over with duct tape to make a ball). It also provides ideas for how to imprint FitBUBBLES with limited access to activity programming (e.g., volunteer at a school's physical education program or recess). This will provide access to different types of activities and the means to engage in activity that is separate from or in addition your FitBASE workout).

APPENDIX B: TEMPLATE IDEAS

The following template ideas are intended to aid your adoption of Iron Footprint Fitness and create your Iron Footprint Icon. The first is a weekly planner to use to ensure that your engagement is intentional and purposeful toward imprinting your Iron Footprint (achieving!), and the second and third are ways to showcase your FitBESTS and FitBUBBLES.

Note - The templates are very primitive! They are meant to help you get *started* organizing your activity engagement as Iron Footprint Fitness and imprinting your Iron Footprint. Hopefully they serve this purpose AND inspire you to create your own that best document the consistency of your FitBASE engagement and showcase your FitBESTS and FitBUBBLES.

Iron Footprint Fitness Weekly Activity Planner

	Cardio	Weights	Stretching	FitBEST Trial	Motor Skill Practice	Novel Activity	Fit BUBBLE	XXXX when done
Monday								
Tuesday								
Wednesday								
Thursday								
Friday								
Saturday								
Sunday								

Iron Footprint Fitness – FitBESTS

- X – FitBESTS that occured during organized events (e.g., running or cycling road races)
- O – FitBESTS that occurred during unorganized events (e.g., during your FitBASE workout)

133

Cardio – X

Event   Date   Result

Cardio - O

Event   Date   Result

Muscular Strength – X

Event   Date   Result

Muscular Strength - O

Event   Date   Result

Muscular Endurance – X

Event   Date   Result

Muscular Endurance – O

Event   Date   Result

Flexibility – X

Event   Date   Result

Flexibility – O

Event   Date   Result

Sports Skills – X

Event   Date   Result

Sports Skills – O

Event   Date   Result

Iron Footprint Fitness FitBUBBLES

A) Each *different* sport/game/activity ever attempted – your clusters

Team Sports	Individual/ Dual Sports	Racquet Activities	Aquatics	Aesthetic Activities	Combatives	Outdoor Activities
-------------	--------------------	-------------	-------------	-------------	---------------	-------------
Basketball	Fencing	Tennis	Swimming	Dance	Karate	Rappelling

Notes: Each category is a 'Universe' (e.g., team sports)
Each Universe may or may not have 'Galaxies' (e.g., basketball is a team sport galaxy)
Each Galaxy may or may not have 'Stars' (e.g., salsa dance is a dance galaxy star)

As your Iron Footprint grows your Universes will become densely populated with Galaxies/Stars

B) Activity separate from/in addition to FitBASE or FitBEST engagement

Date   **Activity**   **Significance (if any)**

Note: These entries may also be entered into your clusters as Universe, Galaxies, or Stars upon your first attempt of them.

APPENDIX C: THE VALUE OF IRON FOOTPRINT FITNESS TO PHYSICAL ACTIVITY INDUSTRY PROFESSIONALS

The Iron Footprint Fitness approach to physical activity offers unique benefit to a wide-range of professionals within the physical activity industry. Physical activity professionals can adopt Iron Footprint Fitness to ensure client/student/athlete success, attract more clients, increase membership or program participation, improve program attendance and retention, underlie the foundation of a program or program-funding proposal, and garner a positive reputation for delivering results. For example, professionals can use IFF to:

- Inspire sales/program registrations by convincing skeptics or nonbelievers how they CAN achieve
- Convey specifics about activity programming to drive a focused conversation
- Enhance program accountability by developing programming intentional to the intended mission

Below is more about Iron Footprint Fitness's value to industry-specific professionals:

Personal Trainers

- Optimize earning and professional reputation:
  - Increase client satisfaction and retention by delivering achievement/nurturing motivation
  - Attract new clients from buzz generated
  - Increase fees – IFF offers added value to a training package
- Compliment the training protocol delivered – adds novelty to workout routines

- Source of professional development – objective performance measures that can be analyzed to determine delivery efficacy, enhanced content knowledge
- Attract new clients who want to adopt Iron Footprint Fitness (join the Iron Footprint Fitness Professional Registry at ironfootprintfitness.com to enhance this effort)

Fitness Managers/Gym Sales Staff/Gym Managers

- Develop a cohesive training stable – we stand for this!
- Incentivize training stable with fitness rather than sales deliverables
- Source of professional development for training stable, enhances content knowledge
- Offer added value to memberships or training packages (IFF will offer ½ off memberships for new or renewed gym members or added training packages/sessions)
- Deal closer– this is how you can realistically achieve and see your achievement – no false claims/guarantees about unrealistic gains
- Create a success-based environment – increased membership/ training services, satisfied clients/members, fewer complaints to respond to, use IFF challenges for gym-wide participation – build morale, positive social media reputation!

Physical Education Teachers

- Create FitBESTS around state learning standards and/or Fitnessgram testing
- Promote/track physical activity outside of class – directly combat childhood obesity
- Focus behavior (purposeful/meaningful class sessions aligned to IFF), reduced off task
- Provide evidence of student learning to students, parents, administrators, school board.

Community-Based Recreation Programs (of programming delivered to all ages – RecreationCenters/Parks, YMCAs, Boys and Girls Clubs, Senior Centers)

- Use to underlie all sports/physical activity programming – creates the thread that runs across all deliverables – this is what we stand for! – and this is what can be expected for each age-group/demographic served, i.e., youth, adult, senior.
- Create a success-based environment which will increase program numbers
- Focus behavior during activities – less off-task
- Provide evidence of program outcomes to participants, parents, local community members, local media, other sites within the system – evidence of combating obesity
- Develop club/facility public displays of members/participants' Footprint, increase club morale and cohesion.
- Create age-appropriate special event programming around FitBESTS and FitBUBBLES

Physical Activity/Physical Education Grant Writers-Fund Seekers

- Provides comprehensive evidence of need, the means to collect data, and outcomes

Coaches (youth, recreation, competitive)

- Sustain effort through specifically focused goals/outcomes (skill development, team play) that the players track
- Create a success-based environment that sustains/increases participation
- Create SPORTPrints specific to your team
- Enhance your reputation as a successful coach

Community-Based Activity/Sport Club Directors (i.e., running clubs, cycling clubs)

- Create a success-based environment that sustains/increases participation/membership
- Create club-based FitBEST or FitBUBBLE challenges to generate excitement and morale
- Create a positive buzz on social media from satisfied club members that attracts new members
- Compile collective group/club Footprint (CLUBprint)

Commercial Fitness Program Owner/Developer (i.e., The Rack, Crossfit, P90x)

- IFF compliments any fitness/exercise program – create/market unique, specific and realistic achievement markers to further entice interested consumers.
- Create a positive buzz on social media specific to users' achievement/satisfaction
- Offer added value to purchase – ½ off IFF membership with purchase

Youth Group Leaders (i.e., Boy/Girl Scouts, church groups)

- Establish a quality physical activity component – create positive pr for combating childhood under-activity, sustain/increase participation/membership – a quality physical activity component WILL draw youth
- Use IFF to frame physical activity programming that fosters attributes of youth development (aligned to the club's intent), show evidence of outcomes/results